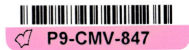

P9-CMV-847

MENTAL HEALTH SERVICES IN THE UNITED STATES AND ENGLAND: STRUGGLING FOR CHANGE

Collected Papers Prepared for The Joint United States/England Conference on Mental Health Services Princeton, New Jersey February 25–28, 1990

Vivian E. Fransen, *Editor*

Special thanks to Barbara Stocking, director of the King's Fund Center, for coordination in England.

A Publication of The Robert Wood Johnson Foundation Communications Office

Thomas P. Gore II, *Vice President for Communications*
Larry Kettelkamp, Victoria D. Weisfeld, *Contributing Editors*
Joan Hollendonner, *Production Coordinator*

Princeton, New Jersey
September 1991

THE ROBERT WOOD JOHNSON FOUNDATION

The Robert Wood Johnson Foundation, the nation's largest private philanthropy devoted to health care issues, was founded as a small, local grantmaker in the mid-1930s by the late General Robert Wood Johnson, who built the Johnson & Johnson family of companies into a major international health and medical care products firm. A national foundation since 1972, it is a private, independent philanthropy unconnected to any corporate interests. More than $1 billion in grants has been awarded since 1972 to improve health care in the United States.

KING EDWARD'S HOSPITAL FUND AND
THE KING'S FUND CENTER

King Edward's Hospital Fund for London is an independent charity founded in 1897 for the support of the hospitals of London. In a wider role today, it stimulates good practice and innovation in all aspects of health care and management through research and development, education, policy analysis, and direct grants. The King's Fund Center is a development agency promoting improvements in health and social care through work with people in health services, social services, voluntary agencies, and their users. It encourages new ideas, provides financial or practical support, and promotes workshops, conferences, and publications. Its aim is to ensure a wider sharing of positive developments in health and social care throughout England.

Library of Congress Catalog Card Number: 91-61190

ISBN 0-942054-03-2

For additional free copies of this publication, write the address below or telephone 609/243-5934.

Communications Office
The Robert Wood Johnson Foundation
Post Office Box 2316
Princeton, NJ 08543-2316

TABLE OF CONTENTS

SECTION I: United States

SECTION II: England

ABOUT THE CONTRIBUTORS: UNITED STATES

Barbara Dickey, PhD, is director of the Mental Health Policy Project at the Massachusetts Mental Health Center in Boston and an assistant professor of psychology at Harvard Medical School. Her expertise is in organization and finance of public mental health systems and in matching outcomes to cost.

Richard G. Frank, PhD, is professor at The Johns Hopkins University and deputy director of the University of Maryland/Johns Hopkins University's Center on Organization and Financing of Care for the Severely Mentally Ill in Baltimore. His research interests lie in the area of economics and mental health.

Howard H. Goldman, MD, PhD, is director of the evaluation study of The Robert Wood Johnson Foundation's Program on Chronic Mental Illness. He is professor of psychiatry at the University of Maryland and director of the mental health policy studies program at the University. He also has extensive experience at the National Institute of Mental Health.

Gerald N. Grob, PhD, is the Henry E. Sigerist Professor of the History of Medicine at Rutgers University. He is the leading historian on the treatment of mental illness in the United States.

Jeffrey C. Merrill is a former vice president of The Robert Wood Johnson Foundation. He has extensive experience in health care policy, especially financing issues, and had oversight responsibility for Foundation programs in areas ranging from the uninsured to mental illness and physical disability.

Herbert Pardes, MD, is vice president for health sciences and dean of the faculty of medicine at the College of Physicians and Surgeons of Columbia University. He is also the president of the American Psychiatric Association (APA) and a past director of the National Institute of Mental Health.

Miles F. Shore, MD, is the program director for The Robert Wood Johnson Foundation's nine-site Program on Chronic Mental Illness. He is also Bullard Professor of Psychiatry at Harvard Medical School, as well as superintendent of the community-based mental health program at the Massachusetts Mental Health Center.

Stephen A. Somers, PhD, is a senior program officer at The Robert Wood Johnson Foundation, who has primary responsibility for a range of programs including the Foundation's Program on Chronic Mental Illness. He has a background in domestic policy at the federal government level.

Leonard I. Stein, MD, is the program director of The Robert Wood Johnson Foundation's Mental Health Services Development Program and is professor of psychiatry at the University of Wisconsin Medical School. He is also the director of research and training at the Mental Health Center of Dane County, which is considered one of the premier community mental health centers in the United States.

ABOUT THE CONTRIBUTORS: ENGLAND

Roger Blunden is director of the community living development team at the King's Fund Center, with an interest in the development of effective community services for people with learning difficulties, mental health problems, and physical disabilities.

Peter Campbell is secretary of Survivors Speak Out. He is currently involved in a World Health Organization initiative on chronic mental illness.

Yvonne Christie is senior project officer for black and mental health services at the King's Fund Center. She has vast experience in working with people who have long-term mental illness. Her main area of concern is development of high quality mental health services reflecting the needs of people from minority racial populations.

Ann Davis is director of social work courses at Birmingham University. She is a trained psychiatric social worker with a strong research interest in social security policy and mental health provision.

Peter Kennedy, MD, was formerly a clinical psychiatrist at Edinburgh University and has published research on the epidemiology of psychiatric disorders. He currently leads a major community care development program in York where he is general manager of all health services for a population of 250,000.

Su Kingsley is service manager of mental health services at Haringey Health Authority in London. She is co-author of the report from the community living development team of the King's Fund Center.

Parimala Moodley is currently employed as director of the Maudsley Outreach Support Team (MOST), a newly formed organization based in Southwark. She is also senior lecturer in community mental health at the Bethlem Royal and Maudsley Hospital in Camberwell, South East London.

Christina Murphy is senior regional planner for mental health, physical disability, and women's and children's services for the North East Thames Regional Health Authority. She was formerly senior development officer at Good Practices in Health, a voluntary organization promoting high quality practices in the mental health field.

Helen Smith is lecturer in mental health at the University of Kent and the regional advisor on mental health services development for the South East Thames Regional Health Authority. She was formerly senior project officer in mental health at the King's Fund.

Simon Whitehead began his career as a social worker. He was formerly first assistant director of Suffolk Social Services and is now deputy director with the National Development Team for people with mental handicaps.

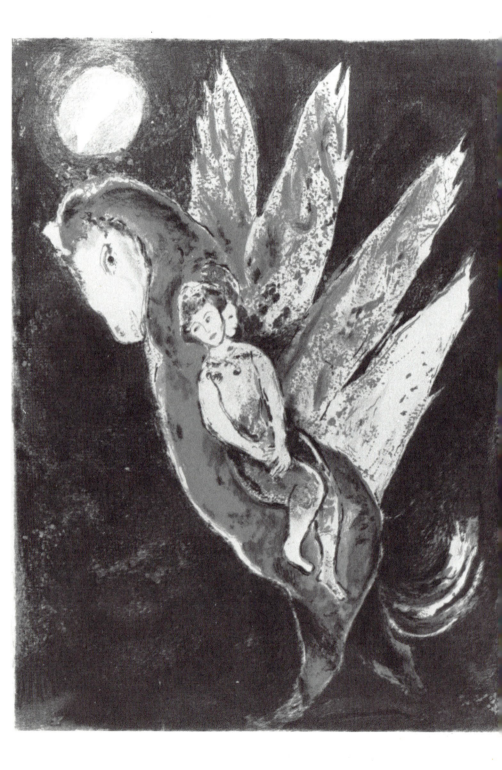

CHRONIC MENTAL ILLNESS IN THE UNITED STATES
An Introduction

By Stephen A. Somers, PhD, and Jeffrey C. Merrill

The Joint United States/England Conference on Mental Health Services came at a propitious time for the American mental health system. As this nation re-examines its overall health care system and its shortcomings in providing access to chronic care services, it is incumbent upon the nation to guarantee adequate coverage to those with serious mental illnesses. Those who work in mental health must be prepared to help improve the efficiency and effectiveness of the mental health system.

In the last several years, The Robert Wood Johnson Foundation has initiated three major programs in the mental health field: the Program on Chronic Mental Illness, the Mental Health Services Development Program, and the Mental Health Services for Youth Program. With evaluations of these programs in progress, it is also a good time for the Foundation to reflect on its investments before considering further steps.

Mental health policy and practice has changed considerably in this country over the past 30 years. The highly visible problems of homeless people with serious mental illnesses have poignantly reinforced the fact that we, as a nation, never completed the task of deinstitutionalization. Although we did establish a series of community-based mental health centers across the country, we never integrated them into a system for the seriously mentally ill. They tend to remain fragmented institutions unevenly committed to serving those with the most severe illnesses. In addition, they were never designed to provide the continuous medical care (e.g., supervision of medication); social support (e.g., care coordination, counseling); or basic life services (e.g., shelter, food) available in a mental hospital. Some professionals in the mental health field have been struggling ever since to fill these gaps. Their goals have been to develop a comprehensive array of community-based services and to rearrange the flow of financing for those services. They have been successful in relatively few locales.

The goal of all three of The Robert Wood Johnson Foundation's major mental health programs is to build community-based systems of care for individuals with serious mental illnesses. While the improvement of mental health services has been at the core of these programs, each has also sought to strengthen related social services, especially housing and psychosocial rehabilitation. In the first of these three efforts, the Program on Chronic Mental Illness, the Foundation enlisted the U.S. Department of Housing and Urban Development as its partner. Together, the agencies have committed approximately $80 million in loans and rent subsidies to generate 3,000–4,000 housing units for adults with serious mental illness.

Each of the programs also directs attention to the critical, but fragmented system of mental health financing in this country. Even though almost all citizens with chronic mental disabilities are supported publicly, few are covered completely by any one source of funds. The only patients whose coverage is comprehensive are those housed in state mental hospitals. For the rest, various governmental programs underwrite health care (Medicaid, state and local mental health programs); income support (supplemental security income for the disabled, welfare); and housing (state mental health programs, federal rent subsidies). The financing is fragmented, inadequate, and hard to get, especially for people with severe mental problems. Too often, it is the local police who eventually bring these displaced individuals back into the service system. Because the fragmentation of our system has been particularly harsh for the seriously mentally ill, many mental health advocates now hold out hope that a more unified health system is imminent in this country and that this population will be one of its prime beneficiaries.

To prepare for this conference, we asked experts on the U.S. mental health system for background papers on the following topics: the history of the system in this country; the dimensions of the problem of chronic mental illness; the organization and financing of mental health services; exemplary services and gaps in the service system; and future directions. These papers provided the basis for much of the discussion at the joint conference supplemented by short formal presentations on other issues such as consumerism and volunteerism, ethnic and minority concerns, and housing and psychosocial rehabilitation. In selecting the U.S. participants, we were also mindful of their additional commitments and expertise in mental health training and research—both of which should be treated as areas of opportunity in the 1990s. The value of these presentations was strengthened by the counterpoint from our English colleagues.

The joint conference has led to this compiled report on the future of community mental health services in both England and the United States. It is hoped that this book will stimulate many who are interested in and dedicated to restructuring the health care system to better meet the complex needs of people with chronic mental illnesses.

∼ THE CHRONIC MENTALLY ILL IN AMERICA:
The Historical Context

By Gerald N. Grob, PhD

In seventeenth- and eighteenth-century America, the problems posed by mental illnesses were relatively minor and of little public concern. Population was sparse, with most individuals living in scattered and somewhat isolated rural and agricultural communities. Hence, the number of mentally ill persons was limited, and they were generally cared for by their families or by local officials who assumed responsibility for their welfare. The mentally ill became a public concern only if they were unable to care for themselves or lacked family connections. They were treated in accordance with the English Poor Law system whose foundations antedated passage of the famous Elizabethan Poor Law legislation written between 1595 and 1601. This system was based on the principle that society had a corporate obligation for poor and dependent persons. Virtually every American colony enacted laws that replicated the English system. Under this arrangement local communities, rather than the colony or mother country, had to assume fiscal and supervisory responsibility for those persons incapable of surviving without some form of assistance.

As a result, before 1800, confinement of the mentally ill was a rare exception rather than the rule. Only when violent behavior threatened others did the community interfere. There was no systematic effort to confine "lunaticks or distracted persons," to use the terminology of the era. Madness was tolerated and family care characteristic. Mentally ill persons without families or private resources received the same treatment as sane paupers; they were either boarded out with families or kept in public almshouses. There was not a clearly defined concept of chronicity, at least not in the medical sense of the term. Insanity became an issue of public concern only when afflicted individuals were unable to secure for themselves the necessities of life. The rural character of American society in the Revolutionary and post-Revolutionary era precluded any serious consideration of structural changes to deal with the mentally ill or other dependent persons.

Origins Of Mental Hospitalization

After 1800, new circumstances ultimately led to reliance on some form of institutional care of the mentally ill. First, demographic changes, including population

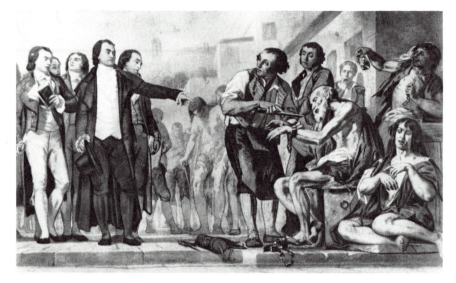

Philippe Pinel (1745–1826) Demanding Removal of Chains from the Insane at the Bicetre Hospital, Paris. Painting by Charles Muller; Courtesy of The Bettmann Archive.

growth, geographic mobility, urbanization, and a rise in immigration, altered the structure of society. Second, a growing awareness of social and medical problems transformed attitudes and perceptions in terms of mental illness. Third, Americans became aware of innovations in France and England as Philippe Pinel's treatise on insanity appeared in 1806 with a wide circulation in the United States, and American Quakers disseminated Samuel Tuke's report on the York Retreat.[1] Finally, religious and intellectual changes, along with a surge in philanthropic giving, stimulated a movement to establish institutions specializing in the care and treatment of the insane. The transformation of insanity into a social problem requiring state intervention in contrast to familial and community responsibility was not a unique phenomenon. The nineteenth century was noted for its widespread use of institutional solutions to social problems and for the transfer of functions from families to public or quasi-public structures. In 1820, only one state hospital for the mentally ill existed in the United States; by the Civil War, virtually every state had established one or more public institutions for that purpose.

Paradoxically, the creation of institutions reflected an extraordinarily optimistic view of the nature and prognosis of mental illness. Most mid-nineteenth-century psychiatrists, influenced by John Locke's concept of the mind as a blank tablet, believed that all knowledge came to the brain through sensory organs. If the senses or the brain were impaired, false impressions would be conveyed to the mind, leading to faulty thinking and abnormal behavior. Mental illness, therefore, was considered a somatic disease that involved lesions of the brain. Such reasoning was especially compatible with a psychological and environmental etiology. Health was assumed to be the consequence of a symbiotic relationship among nature, society, and the individual. As such, it was synonymous with order and virtue. Disease, on the other hand, followed the violation of the natural laws that governed human nature and was indissolubly linked with immorality and improper living conditions. Since insanity was the result of improper behavioral patterns associated with a defective environment, therapy had to begin with the creation of a new and presumably more appropriate environment. Home treatment was useless, for the physician had no means of eliminating undesirable environmental influences. Institutionalization was a *sine qua non* because it shattered the link between an improper environment and the patient. In a hospital, patients could be exposed to both medical and moral treatment. Medical treatment was intended to rebuild the body, to improve the moral state, and to calm violent behavior by the administration of narcotics. "Moral treatment" implied kind, individualized care within a small hospital utilizing occupational therapy and resorting to religious exercises, amusements, and games. There were to be no threats of physical violence, and only rarely were mechanical means of restraint to be employed. Moral treatment, in effect, involved the reeducation of the patient within a more suitable environment. The role of the psychiatrist was not fundamentally different from the role of the stern yet loving and concerned father.

Curability And Chronicity In The Nineteenth Century

From the prevailing model of disease, psychiatrists drew an obvious conclusion that insanity was at least as curable as most somatic illnesses. "Insanity," proclaimed Samuel B. Woodward in 1839, first president of what is now the American Psychiatric Association (APA), "of all diseases the most fearful, is found to be among the most curable."[2] It was common for mental hospital superintendents in the 1830s and 1840s to claim that 90 percent or more of all recent cases defined as being insane for one year or less could be cured if treated promptly. William M. Awl, a contemporary of Woodward and superintendent of the Ohio Lunatic Asylum, reported that, in the first four years following its opening in 1838, it had received 171 persons insane for one year or less; 69 between one and two years; 85 between two and five years; and 44 between five and ten years. Recovery rates within each group were 80, 35, 14, and nine percent, respectively.[3] Within such an intellectual framework, the concept of chronicity had a somewhat different meaning. Chronicity was neither inherent nor inevitable, but followed the failure to provide acute cases with the benefit of therapy in mental hospitals. "The incurable insane," wrote Edward Jarvis in 1855, remain standing and abiding monuments of the neglect of the State to provide the means of health, and place them within the reach or the comprehension of the friends and guardians who had immediate charge of them, or of the neglect of those friends and guardians to avail themselves of these opportunities of restoration when they were offered to them.[4]

Psychiatrists, moreover, denied that a recurrence of insanity was simply a continuation of the original illness. Just as individuals could suffer numerous respiratory or intestinal diseases, so, too, could they have subsequent unrelated episodes of insanity. Woodward, for example, argued that if a patient discharged as recovered had been free of symptoms for a year or more, any recurrence was attributable to a new cause that had no relation to the previous attack. He said that if individuals who recovered would avoid "known causes of disease . . . they might safely pass on, and, in most cases, continue well." "It is just as possible," observed Thomas S. Kirkbride in his classic work on mental hospitals, "for anyone to have an attack of insanity, to recover from it, and to have another attack at a subsequent period of life, as it is of any other disease, or as any one is liable to have a first attack."[5]

In general, patients discharged as recovered or improved tended to be institutionalized for only brief periods from three to nine months. Hence the prevailing belief was that a mental hospital with 200 beds could treat approximately 600 patients during a twelve-month period, assuming that the average stay would be about four months. Surviving evidence suggests that the claims of therapeutic successes had some validity. Although affirmations about curability rates were undoubtedly exaggerated, there is little doubt that many individuals appeared to have benefited from hospitalization. In the 1880s, an enterprising superintendent undertook a follow-up study of over a thousand patients discharged as recovered. The study took more than a decade to complete, and in the end, data were accumulated on 984 individuals. Of these, 317 were alive and well, while an additional 251 had died but had never again been institutionalized. Thus, nearly 58 percent of those discharged as recovered had functioned in a community setting without any relapse.[6]

The absence of a large chronic institutional population further reinforced the faith in curability. Between the 1830s and 1870s, the proportion of long-term or chronic cases in hospitals was relatively low—that is, if the figures are compared with the extraordinarily high percentage between 1890 and 1950. Although national data are lacking, a sample of individual hospitals reveals that their functions as custodial institutions had not yet become dominant. The experiences of Worcester State Hospital, the oldest and most important public institution in Massachusetts, were instructive. In 1842, a decade after it opened, 46.4 percent of its patients had been hospitalized for less than a year, while only 13.2 percent had been in the hospital for five or more years. In 1870, the comparable figures were 49.6 and 13.9 percent. Nor was Worcester atypical. In 1850, 41.4 percent of the patients at the Virginia Western Lunatic Asylum had been hospitalized for less than a year and 29.6 percent for five years or more. The respective figures for the California Insane Asylum in 1860 were 40.2 and 0.1. Unlike their twentieth-century counterparts, hospitals before 1880 did not have many aged patients (over 65) or paretics, those in the tertiary stage of syphilis. Between 1830 and 1875, aged patients accounted for only about five to 10 percent of the total. In the Utica Hospital, only 2.7 percent of all admissions between 1850 and 1868 were afflicted with general paresis.[7]

The low proportion of chronic patients in mental hospitals was due partly to the pattern of funding. In general, state legislatures provided the capital funds necessary for acquiring new sites and constructing, expanding, and renovating existing physical plants, whereas local communities were required to pay hospitals a sum equal to the actual cost of care and treatment of each patient admitted. The system, moreover, did not assume that every mentally ill person would be cared for in a state institution. Laws generally required that only dangerous mentally ill persons had to be sent to state hospitals. Others who would presumably benefit from therapeutic interventions could, at the discretion of local officials, also be institutionalized. The system, in short, involved divided responsibility.

For much of the nineteenth century, a significant proportion of persons considered insane continued either to live in the community or were kept in municipal almshouses. Families with sufficient resources could commit their relatives to state institutions, provided they were willing to assume financial liability for their upkeep. States had to reimburse hospitals for those patients who had not established legal residency, such as immigrants. The result was a variegated pattern. Edward Jarvis's census of all persons identified by others as insane in Massachusetts in 1854 provides some insight into the distribution of the mentally ill. In his monumental survey, Jarvis identified, by name, every such person in the Bay State. According to his final tabulations, there were 2,632 persons designated insane. Of this number, 1,522 were paupers, and 1,110 were supported by their own resources or by friends. At the time, 1,284 were either at home or in almshouses; 1,141 were in hospitals; and 207 were in local receptacles for the insane, houses of correction, jails, or state almshouses. Only 435 were identified as curable, as compared with 2,018 incurable (the prognosis of 179 was unknown).[8]

Divided responsibility for the mentally ill had significant repercussions. The system tended to promote competition and rivalries between overlapping governmental jurisdictions. In many states the stipulation that individual communities were financially liable for their poor and indigent insane residents created incentives for local officials to keep them in almshouses where costs were lower. Hospital officials often faced unremitting pressure from communities to discharge patients regardless of their condition in order to save money. Local officials on occasion even attempted to force hospitals to reimburse the community for work performed by patients even though such labor was part of a therapeutic regimen. Ironically, divided fiscal and government authority had the paradoxical effect of keeping the chronic population in mental hospitals at relatively low levels.

Mid-nineteenth-century psychiatrists generally opposed the establishment of separate institutions for chronic or incurable cases, and accepted the legitimacy of custodial care. They were not certain if they could distinguish between curable and incurable cases and feared that the prevention of custodial abuse would be overly difficult. Moreover, their experiences with local officials led them to conclude that confinement of the chronic insane in almshouses or comparable institutions was detrimental. In the first edition of his classic work, Kirkbride vigorously condemned the maintenance of chronic patients in separate institutions and insisted that all insane persons required identical care. When he published a second edition of his work a quarter of a century later, his views had not changed. "What is best for the recent," he insisted, "is best for the chronic."[9]

The Rise Of Chronicity

As the number of chronic patients increased, states slowly began to reconsider their policies. Massachusetts and New York, which maintained the most extensive hospital systems, introduced some significant modifications. In the 1850s, Massachusetts created a separate department for chronic insane immigrants at its state almshouse. In 1869, New York opened the Willard Asylum, which was intended to relieve local welfare institutions of any responsibility for poor chronic insane patients. By the 1880s, Wisconsin established a controversial system that provided state subsidies for the care of chronic cases at county-run facilities. These and other policy innovations had two distinct goals: to ensure that hospitals retained their therapeutic character and to minimize the role of local communities whose officials were preoccupied with maintaining low tax rates. The effort to segregate the chronic population met with an ambivalent reception from psychiatrists. Senior figures opposed a policy that stigmatized large numbers of individuals and consigned them to custodial institutions. Those in favor of the new departure argued that the retention of chronic patients in local poorhouses institutionalized an inferior system.

The debate over a policy that divided curable and chronic cases was basically rendered moot by the turn of the century. Disillusioned by a system that divided authority, states—led once again by New York and Massachusetts—adopted legislation that relieved local communities of any role whatsoever in caring for the mentally ill. The assumption of those who favored centralization was that local care, although less expensive, was substandard and also fostered chronicity and dependency. Conversely, care and treatment in hospitals, though more costly initially, would in the long run be cheaper, because it would enhance recovery for some and provide more humane care for others.

Although the intent of state assumption of responsibility was to ensure that the mentally ill would receive a higher quality of care and treatment, the consequences turned out to be quite different, as local officials saw a golden opportunity to shift some of their financial obligations onto the state. The purpose of the state care legislation was self-evident, namely, to remove the care of the chronically mentally ill from local jurisdictions. But local officials went beyond the intent of the law. Traditionally, nineteenth-century almshouses supported and administered by local government served, in part, as homes for senile and aged persons who had no financial resources. The passage of state care acts provided local officials with an unexpected opportunity. They redefined senility in psychiatric terms and began to transfer aged people from local almshouses to state mental hospitals. Humanitarian concerns played a relatively minor role in this development; economic considerations were paramount.

Faced with rapidly escalating expenditures, communities were happy to transfer responsibility for their aged residents to state-supported facilities. Therefore, between 1880 and 1920 the almshouse populations, for this and other reasons, dropped precipitously. Admissions fell from 99.5 to 58.4 per 100,000 population between 1904 and 1922. At the same time the general decline reported in the number of mentally ill persons aged 60 and over was even sharper, dropping from 24.3 percent in 1880 to 5.6 percent in 1923.[10] What occurred, however, was not a deinstitutionalization movement, but rather a lateral transfer of individuals from one institution to another. "We are receiving every year a large number of old people, some of them very old, who are simply suffering from the mental decay incident to extreme old age," observed Charles C. Wagner, superintendent of the Binghampton State Hospital in New York.

> A little mental confusion, forgetfulness and garrulity are sometimes the only symptoms exhibited, but the patient is duly certified to us as insane and has no one at home capable or possessed of means to care for him. We are unable to refuse these patients without creating ill-feeling in the community where they reside, nor are we able to assert that they are not insane within the meaning of the statute, for many of them, judged by the ordinary standards of sanity, cannot be regarded as entirely sane.[11]

During the first half of the twentieth century, as a result, the character of mental hospitals underwent a dramatic transformation. Prior to that time, hospitals had substantial turnover rates even though they retained patients who failed to improve or recover. In the four decades following the opening of the Utica State Lunatic Asylum in the 1840s, the proportion of patients who left the institution hovered around 40 percent. In the twentieth century, by way of contrast, the pattern changed markedly as the proportion of short-term cases fell and that of long-term increased. In 1904, 27.8 percent of the total mental patient population in the United States had been institutionalized for twelve months or less. By 1910, this percentage fell to 12.7, although it rose to 17.4 in 1923. The greatest change, however, came among patients hospitalized for five years or more. In 1904, 39.2 percent of patients fell into this category; in 1910 and 1923, the respective percentages were 52.0 and 54.0. Although data for the United States as a whole were unavailable after 1923, the experiences of Massachusetts are illustrative. By the 1930s nearly 80 percent of its mental hospital beds were occupied by chronic patients.[12]

Chronicity, however, is a somewhat misleading term, for the group that it described was actually heterogeneous. Those 60 years or older constituted, by far, the single largest component. By 1920, for example, 18 percent of all first admissions to New York state mental hospitals were diagnosed as psychotic because of senility or arteriosclerosis. Twenty years later, the figure had risen to 31 percent. A decade later, 40 percent of all first admissions were aged 60 and over, as compared with only 13.2 percent of the state's total population. The increase in the absolute number also reflected a change in age-specific admission rates. In their classic study on rates of institutionalization covering more than a century, Goldhamer and Marshall found that the greatest increase occurred in the older category. In 1855, the age-specific first-admission rate in Massachusetts aged 60 and over was 70.4 for males and 65.5 for females (per 100,000); by the beginning of World War II, the corresponding figures were 279.5 and 223.0. As late as 1958, nearly a third of all resident state hospital patients were over 65.[13]

The rising age of distribution mirrored a different but related characteristic of the institutionalized; namely, the presence of many patients whose abnormal behavior reflected a somatic etiology. Even allowing for imprecise diagnoses and an imperfect statistical reporting system, it was evident that a significant proportion of the hospitalized population suffered from severe organic disorders for which there were no effective treatments. Of 49,116 first admitted in 1922 because of various psychoses, 16,407 suffered from a variety of identifiable somatic conditions, such as senility, cerebral arteriosclerosis, paresis, Huntington's chorea, and brain tumors. Between 1922 and 1940, the proportion of such patients increased from 33.4 to 42.4 percent. In 1946, various forms of senility and paresis accounted for about half of all first admissions.[14]

Creation Of New Community Policies

By the mid-1940s, it had become clear that mental hospitals had been transformed by the nature of their patient populations. The presence of so many aged persons and others suffering from irreversible somatic disorders signified that institutions were providing custodial care for those who would remain there until they died. A study of 683 aged persons admitted to Maryland hospitals in the early 1940s revealed that 47 percent died within the first year and overall, only 10 percent were ever discharged.[15]

In the immediate postwar years, journalists and mental health professionals published numerous critical accounts of mental hospitals, even though their analyses were not always accurate. Admittedly, a decade and a half of financial neglect, due largely to the combined impact of the Great Depression of the 1930s and global conflict of the 1940s, simply exacerbated already existing severe problems. The depressing state of mental hospitals, however, was as much a function of the nature of their patients as it was the result of parsimonious or callous policies. The large number of chronically ill patients was undoubtedly the single most significant element in failing to accomplish therapeutic goals.

Mental hospitals which had been the cornerstone of public policy for nearly a century and a half began to lose their social and medical legitimacy. This was hardly surprising. After World War II, the prevailing consensus on mental health policy slowly began to dissolve. A number of developments converged to reshape public policy during these years. First, psychiatric thinking shifted toward a psychodynamic and psychoanalytic model emphasizing life experiences and socioenvironmental factors. Second, the experiences of World War II appeared to demonstrate the efficacy of community and outpatient treatment of disturbed persons. Third, the belief that early intervention in the community would be effective in preventing subsequent hospitalization became popular. Fourth, a faith developed that psychiatry could promote prevention by ameliorating social problems that allegedly fostered mental diseases. Fifth, the introduction of psychological and somatic therapies (including, but not limited to, psychotropic drugs) held out the promise of a more normal existence for patients outside of mental institutions. Finally, an enhanced social welfare role of the federal government not only began to diminish the authority of state governments, but also hastened the transition from an institutionally-based to a community-oriented policy.

Winds of change were evident well before the widespread use of psychotropic drugs or the advent of deinstitutionalization. The specialty of psychiatry, long synonymous with institutional care, rapidly changed its character in the postwar era. To be sure, psychiatrists began to find careers outside public institutions in the interwar decades. But after 1945, there was a mass exodus of psychiatrists from mental hospitals into private and community practice. Within a decade, more than 80 percent of the 10,000 members of the APA were employed outside of mental hospitals. Their positions were filled by foreign medical graduates with little or no training in psychiatry.[16] Although the APA staff continued to work with public hospitals, especially through the Central Inspection Board and annual Mental Hospital Institutes, most of its members were neither knowledgeable about nor sympathetic toward their institutional counterparts and often emphasized the desirability of noninstitutional alternatives. Most psychiatrists in the community treated large numbers of patients with psychological problems, thus sharply reducing their contact with the severely mentally ill. The large proportion of chronic patients in hospitals hardly accorded with the self-image of the psychiatrist as an active and successful therapist. In his APA presidential address in 1958, Harry C. Solomon even described the large mental hospital as "antiquated, outmoded, and rapidly becoming obsolete." Robert C. Hunt, director of the Hudson River State Hospital in New York and an individual deeply concerned with institutional problems, responded publicly in critical terms. His "private reactions are still unprintable," he wrote to Solomon. Hunt subsequently informed the APA Commission on Long-Term Planning that the organization had not played a constructive role in countering the detrimental effects associated with "the state hospital stereotype." The majority of APA members, he added, had neither the contacts with nor knowledge about mental hospitals. Hence, its members were prone to identify the prevailing stereotype with reality; the result was a virtual abandonment of the hospital by American psychiatrists.[17]

The weakening of the long-established links between hospitals and psychiatrists was also accompanied by a movement to strengthen outpatient and community clinics. Before 1940, such clinics had dealt predominantly with children rather than adults. The postwar enthusiasm for clinics received momentum with the passage of the National Mental Health Act of 1946, which provided grants to states to support existing outpatient facilities or to establish new ones. The ultimate goal, according to Robert H. Felix, first director of the National Institute for Mental Health (NIMH), was one outpatient facility for each 100,000 persons. Although appropriations were modest, the impact of these clinics was dramatic. Before 1948, more than half of all states had no clinics; by 1949, all but five had one or more. Six years later, there were about 1,234 outpatient psychiatric clinics, of which about two-thirds were state supported or aided. Psychiatrists proved staunch proponents of a community-oriented policy, for they insisted that early identification and treatment in outpatient facilities or private offices diminished the need for subsequent hospitalization and were cost effective as well.[18]

During the 1950s, support for a community-based policy increased steadily. The Governor's Conference and Council of State Governments, as well as private foundations such as the Milbank Memorial Fund, played important roles in marshaling support for innovation. In 1954, New York enacted its influential Community Mental Health Services Act, which provided state funding for outpatient clinics. California followed suit shortly thereafter with the passage of the Short-Doyle Act. By 1959, there were more than 1,400 clinics serving about 502,000 individuals, of whom 294,000 were over the age of eighteen.[19] The expansion of community facilities was accompanied by the availability of new services to schools, courts, and social agencies provided by nonmedical mental health professionals. This development offered further proof of the degree to which the public sought access to psychiatric and psychological services in noninstitutional settings. During these years, Robert Felix and his NIMH colleagues worked with key congressional figures to enhance the policymaking authority of the federal government as a vehicle to strengthen community policies.

Many of the claims about the efficacy of community care and treatment, however, rested on extraordinarily shaky foundations. The presumption was that outpatient psychiatric clinics could identify early cases of mental disorders and also serve as alternatives to mental hospitals. The empirical data to validate such assertions, however, were lacking. A study of about 500 patients in three California state hospitals during the 1950s found most of them unsuited to treatment in clinics. The authors concluded by noting "the marked discontinuities in functions of the participating hospitals and clinics and the difficulties in initiating outpatient treatment with hospitalized patients shortly after their admission." They also called attention to "the value of services to bridge the gap between the traditional functions of hospitals and clinics for already hospitalized patients."[20] Data collected by Morton Kramer and his associates at the Biometrics Branch of NIMH raised equally serious questions. A community policy was based on the expectation that patients could be treated outside of institutions. Underlying this belief were several assumptions: that patients had a home and a sympathetic family or other person willing and able to assume responsibility for their care; that the organization of their household would aid rehabilitation; and that the patient's presence would not cause undue hardship for other family members. In 1960, however, 48 percent of the mental hospital population was unmarried, 12 percent was widowed, and 13 percent was divorced or separated. A large proportion of patients may have had no families to care for them. Hence, the assumption that patients could reside in the community with their families while undergoing rehabilitation was hardly realistic.[21]

Such findings fell on deaf ears. The rubric of community care and treatment carried the day in the 1950s and 1960s. Too often exaggerated claims have been overlooked or ignored. Such rhetoric has shaped agendas and debates; created expectations that, in turn, molded policies; and shaped the socialization, training, and education of those in professional occupations. From the creation of the Joint Commission on Mental Illness and Health in 1955 and the publication of its influential *Action for Mental Health: Final Report of the Joint Commission on Mental Illness and Health 1961* to the passage of the Community Mental Health Centers Act of 1963, the advocates of a community-oriented policy succeeded in forging a consensus regarding the desirability of diminishing the central role of mental hospitals while strengthening community facilities. These advocates were joined by a variety of other individuals and groups. Psychiatric critics attacked the very legitimacy of the concept of mental illness. Civil rights advocates identified the mentally ill as a group systematically deprived of constitutional liberties; and social activists emphasized that institutions such as mental hospitals are inherently repressive and dehumanizing. The result was a determined and partially successful effort to reshape public policy by diminishing the role of hospitals and enhancing the significance of outpatient and community services.

During the 1960s, the attack on the legitimacy of institutional care began to bear fruit. Hospital populations declined rapidly after 1965. A shift in thinking had made community care and treatment, at least in theory, an acceptable alternative to institutionalization. Administrative and structural changes within institutions, including open-door policies, informal admissions, and efforts to prepare patients for early release, as well as the introduction of psychotropic drugs, reinforced the faith in the efficacy of community treatment. The passage of Medicaid and Medicare legislation hastened the exodus of elderly patients from hospitals to nursing homes. The rapid expansion of third-party reimbursement plans stimulated the use of inpatient and outpatient psychiatric services in general hospitals. Ironically, the reduction of the psychiatric hospital patient population with accompanying improvement in patient/staff ratio no doubt had the effect of improving the lives of those who remained in public mental hospitals.

In conclusion, the consequences of human activities tend to be complex and unpredictable; ambiguity instead of clarity or consistency is often characteristic. This is especially true for the changes in the mental health system since World War II. Prior to 1940, public policy had been focused almost exclusively on the severely and chronically mentally ill. This policy was based on the assumption that society had an obligation to provide such unfortunate persons with both care and treatment in public mental hospitals. The policies adopted during and after the 1960s rested on quite different assumptions. Public mental hospitals continued to play an important role, but the creation of a decentralized heterogeneous system of services diminished their relative significance. Equally important, the target population became more diffuse and variegated so that policymakers of the mental health system were no longer concerned solely with the severely and chronically mentally ill. Even those professionals involved in providing services were less likely to deal specifically with individuals with severe mental illness who presented formidable and sometimes insoluble problems. Ironically, the growing availability, variety, and popularity of mental health services then sometimes worked to the detriment of this subgroup most in need of assistance.

Perhaps one of the most striking results of the postwar shift in policy was the breaking of the traditional and hitherto inseparable ties between care and treatment. Despite monumental shortcomings, mental hospitals had provided at least a basic level of care for many individuals incapable of functioning as independent and self-reliant human beings. Moreover, mental hospital care had derived legitimacy from its identification with medical science. Thus, these institutions did not have to bear the burden of being tied to a welfare system grounded in part on the belief that dependency was self-inflicted, and that poverty, misfortune, and illness were consequences of character deficiencies rather than environmental or biological circumstances.

The community mental health policies that emerged during the postwar decades inadvertently distorted priorities by strengthening the distinction between care and treatment. Admittedly, these policies paid lip service to the need for care. The reality, however, was quite different. The main focus was on providing therapeutic services in outpatient settings to a broad rather than a narrowly defined population. Consequently, the social and human needs of the most severely chronically mentally ill, particularly assistance in dealing with the subsistence tasks of daily life, were often ignored or overlooked. The identification of mental health policy with therapeutic services was understandable, given the obvious advantages of being included within the medical health care system. Caring and support services, by contrast, were affiliated with a welfare system that, by the 1970s and 1980s, was under attack by a political constituency bent on diminishing governmental responsibilities and activities.

The subtle shifts in the mental health system were to have tragic consequences for many chronically and severely mentally ill persons most in need of assistance. In the 1970s and 1980s, they were often cast adrift in communities without access to support services or the basic necessities of life. For many, the transition from an institutional to a community-based system proved devastating. By the 1980s, the presence of homeless mentally ill persons served as a stark reminder that the new mental health policies had negative as well as positive consequences.[22]

Notes

The research for this paper was supported by a grant from the National Institute for Mental Health (MH39030); Public Health Service; U.S. Department of Health and Human Services. Many of the data and generalizations are taken from my previous books, *Mental Institutions in America: Social Policy to 1875* (New York, 1973), *Mental Illness and American Society, 1975–1950* (Princeton, 1983), and *From Asylum to Community: Mental Health Policy in Modern America* (Princeton, 1991).

1. Philippe Pinel, *A Treatise on Insanity* (Sheffield, England, 1806); and Samuel Tuke, *Description of the Retreat, an Institution Near York for Insane Persons of the Society of Friends* (York, England, 1813).
2. Worcester State Lunatic Hospital, *Annual Report 7* (1839), 65.
3. Ohio Lunatic Asylum, *Annual Report 4* (1842), 57.
4. *Report on Insanity and Idiocy in Massachusetts by the Commission on Lunacy Under Resolve of the Legislature of 1854* (Massachusetts *House Document No. 144* [1855]: Boston: William White, 1855), 70.
5. Worcester State Lunatic Hospital, *Annual Report 8* (1840), 47; 9 (1841), 68; 10 (1842), 62; Thomas S. Kirkbride, *On the Construction, Organization, and General Arrangements of Hospitals for the Insane* (original ed. 1854; second ed., Philadelphia, 1880), 23.
6. Worcester State Lunatic Hospital, *Annual Report 61* (1893), 70.
7. Worcester State Lunatic Hospital, *Annual Report 10* (1842), 17–27; 25 (1857), 55–56; 34 (1866), 67; 35 (1867), 34; 38 (1870), 38–60; Virginia Western Lunatic Asylum, *Annual Report 23* (1850), 14–23; California Insane Asylum, *Annual Report 8* (1860), 16–32; Insane Asylum of Louisiana, *Annual Report* (1858), 13; New York City Lunatic Asylum, Blackwell's Island, *Annual Report* (1861), 17; New Hampshire Asylum for the Insane, *Annual Report 23* (1864), 16; Utica State Lunatic Asylum, *Annual Report 38* (1870), 18–19; Western Pennsylvania Hospital, *Annual Report* (1871), 18–19.
8. *Report on Insanity and Idiocy*, 18, 73. All of the manuscript returns listing every person by name can be found in "Report of the Physicians of Massachusetts. Superintendents of Hospitals . . . and Others Describing the Insane and Idiotic Persons in the State of Massachusetts in 1855, Made to the Commissioners on Lunacy," manuscript volume in the Countway Library of Medicine, Harvard Medical School, Boston, Massachusetts.
9. Kirkbride, first ed., 59, second ed., 248.
10. Data on almshouse populations are drawn from the following U.S. Bureau of

the Census publications: *Paupers in Almshouses 1904* (Washington, D.C., 1906), 182, 184; *Paupers in Almshouses 1910* (Washington, D.C., 1915), 42–43; *Paupers in Almshouses 1923* (Washington, D.C., 1925), 5, 8, 33; *Insane and Feeble-Minded in Hospitals and Institutions 1904* (Washington, D.C., 1906), 29; *Patients in Hospitals for Mental Diseases 1923* (Washington, D.C., 1926), 7.

11. New York State Commission on Lunacy, *Annual Report* 12(1900), 29–30.

12. Ellen Dwyer, *Homes for the Mad: Life Inside Two Nineteenth-Century Asylums* (New Brunswick, 1987), 150–151; *Insane and Feeble-Minded in Hospitals and Institutions 1904*, 37; U.S. Bureau of the Census, *Insane and Feeble-Minded in Institutions 1910* (Washington, D.C., 1914), 59; *Patients in Hospitals for Mental Disease 1923*, 36; Neil A. Dayton, *New Facts on Mental Disorders: Study of 89,190 Cases* (Springfield, Ill., 1940), 414–429.

13. Benjamin Malzberg, "A Statistical Analysis of the Ages of First Admissions to Hospitals for Mental Disease in New York State," *Psychiatric Quarterly* 20 (1949), 344–366; Ibid. "A Comparison of First Admissions to the New York Civil State Hospitals During 1919–1921 and 1949–1951," Ibid. 28 (1954), 312–319; New York State Department of Mental Hygiene, *Annual Report* 42 (1939–1940), 174–175; Herbert Goldhamer and Andrew W. Marshall, *Psychosis and Civilization: Two Studies in the Frequency of Mental Disease* (Glencoe, Ill., 1953), 54, 91; American Psychiatric Association, *Report on Patients Over 65 in Public Mental Hospitals* (Washington, D.C., 1960), 5.

14. Statistics compiled from U.S. Bureau of the Census, *Patients in Hospitals for Mental Disease 1923, Mental Patients in State Hospitals 1926 and 1927* (Washington, D.C., 1930); *Patients in Mental Hospitals 1940* (Washington, D.C., 1943); and Morton Kramer, *Psychiatric Services and the Changing Institutional Scene, 1950–1985* (DHEW Publication No. [ADM] 76—374 (Washington, D.C., 1976), 75.

15. Oswaldo Camargo and George H. Preston, "What Happens to Patients Who Are Hospitalized for the First Time When Over Sixty-Five Years of Age?" *American Journal of Psychiatry*, 102 (1945), 168–173.

16. Data on the location of psychiatrists taken from the following: *Biographical Directory of Fellows & Members of the American Psychiatric Association as of October 1, 1957* (New York, 1958); "Distribution of Members of the American Psychiatric Association 1910–1960," Miscellaneous Papers, Box 1, Archives of the APA, Washington, D.C.; Joint Information Service, *Fact Sheet No. 2* (May, 1957) and *No. 10* (August, 1959), David A. Boyd, "Current and Future Trends in Psychiatric Residency Training," *Journal of Medical Education*, 33 (1958): 345–346.

17. Harry C. Solomon, "The American Psychiatric Association in Relation to American Psychiatry," *American Journal of Psychiatry*, 115 (1958), 1–9; *New York Times*, May 13, 16, 1958; Robert C. Hunt to Solomon, June 17, Solomon to Hunt, June 19, 1958, Solomon Papers, Archives of the APA; Robert C. Hunt, "The State Hospital Stereotype" (statement before the APA Commission on Long-term Planning, October 30, 1959); Records of the Medical Director's Office, Archives of the APA, 200–11.

18. *New York Times*, April 4, 1947; NIMH, "Annual Report, Fiscal 1949," 9–10; NIMH Records, Subject Files, 1940–51, Box 82, Washington National Records Center, Suitland, Maryland; Anita K. Bahn and Vivian B. Norman, *Outpatient Psychiatric Clinics in the United States 1954–55* (U.S. Public Health Service *Public Health Monograph 49*: Washington, D.C., 1957), 38.

19. "Gains in Outpatient Psychiatric Services, 1959," *Public Health Report*, 75 (1960), 1092–1094; Vivian B. Norman, Beatrice M. Rosen, and Anita K. Bahn, "Psychiatric Clinic Outpatients in the United States, 1959," *Mental Hygiene*, 46 (1962), 321–343.

20. Harold Sampson, David Ross, Bernice Engle, and Florine Livson, "Feasibility of Community Clinic Treatment for State Mental Hospital Patients," *Archives of Neurology and Psychiatry*, 80 (1958), 77. A larger version of this study appeared under the title *A Study of Suitability for Outpatient Clinic Treatment of State Mental Hospital Admissions 1957*, California Department of Mental Hygiene, *Research Report No. 1* (1957).

21. See Morton Kramer, *Some Implications of Trends in the Usage of Psychiatric Facilities for Community Mental Health Programs and Related Research* (U.S. Public Health Service *Publication 1434*:1967); Ibid. "Epidemiology, Biostatistics, and Mental Health Planning," APA *Psychiatric Research Reports*, 22 (1967), 1–68; Kramer, C. Taube, and S. Starr, "Patterns of Use of Psychiatric Facilities by the Aged: Current Status, Trends, and Implications," APA *Psychiatric Research Reports*, 23 (1968), 89–150.

22. See H. Richard Lamb, ed., *The Homeless Mentally Ill: A Task Force Report of the American Psychiatric Association* (Washington, D.C., 1984).

∿ THE DIMENSIONS OF THE CHALLENGE

By Miles F. Shore, MD, and Barbara Dickey, PhD

On January 23, 1751, Benjamin Franklin and a group of concerned citizens petitioned the Pennsylvania Assembly for assistance in creating what would become the Pennsylvania Hospital. In the document, Franklin and his associates made this case:

> That with the numbers of people, the number of lunaticks, or persons distempered in mind, and deprived of their rational faculties, hath greatly increased in this Province.
>
> That some of them going at large, are a terrour to their neighbors, who are daily apprehensive of the violences they may commit; and others are continually wasting their substance, to the great injury of themselves and families, ill disposed persons wickedly taking advantage of their unhappy condition, and drawing them into unreasonable bargains etc.
>
> That few or none of them are so sensible of their condition as to submit voluntarily to the treatment their respective cases require, and therefore continue in the same deplorable state during their lives; whereas it has been found by the experience of many years, that above two thirds of the mad people received into Bethlehem Hospital, and there treated properly, have been perfectly cured.[1]

The antique language cloaks a problem with familiar dimensions. Substantial numbers of persons are afflicted with mental illness. There are associated costs to individuals and society, such as threats to public order; both real and imagined exploitation of the vulnerable; and the special provisions required for persons whose illnesses affect their capacity to seek effective treatment.

Defining Chronic Mental Illness

Current definitions of chronic mental illness (CMI) are based on diagnosis, degree of disability, and duration. There is disagreement about each of these features.

In an effort to identify those with chronic mental illness, the Department of Health and Human Services (DHHS) Steering Committee on CMI reported that the largest group, from 35–52 percent of those with chronic mental illness, is comprised of persons with organic brain syndrome, severe character disorder, and other conditions. From 29–37 percent have schizophrenia, while major affective disorders account for 33–35 percent.[2] More recent consideration suggests that any conditions severe enough to lead to disability should be included within the CMI rubric.[3]

Disability involves the inability to function in major aspects of life, such as self-care, learning, independent living, social relationships, and economic self-sufficiency. To establish eligibility for Supplemental Security Income (SSI/SSDI), the Social Security Administration restricts its definition to the inability to engage in any substantial gainful activity due to a disorder which has lasted or can be expected to last for a continuous period of not less than 12 months.

The duration of the illness was easier to determine when the majority of persons with CMI were hospitalized for long periods of time. Traditional definitions required a continuous period of hospitalization of at least 12 months. In recognition of deinstitutionalization, the definition was expanded by the National Institute of Mental Health (NIMH) Community Support Program to include either a single episode of hospitalization of at least six months duration in the last five years or two or more hospitalizations within a 12-month period. Unfortunately, this definition includes persons with any mental disorder, even a relatively mild one, who may have had two acute episodes or a brief relapse from a first episode within a year. It also excludes the large number of persons who are severely impaired by mental illness but are kept out of a hospital by community alternatives.

Where once the length of stay for hospitalized mental patients could be reported in months or years, today the length of stay is relatively brief. At one time the NIMH Division of Biometry and Epidemiology considered patients who stayed longer than 90 days to be chronically mentally ill. However, today 80 percent are discharged sooner. This illustrates the flaw in establishing duration of disability by the amount or extent of treatment received rather than simply by the length of time of impairment. Hospitalization persists as a de facto criterion of CMI because it is clearly definable. As L. L. Bachrach has pointed out in her concept paper on CMI, there are serious, practical consequences when hospitalization is used as a standard for eligibility for disability benefits.[4]

In their 1981 review of this matter, H. H. Goldman and his associates have offered the following definition:

> The chronically mentally ill population encompasses persons who suffer certain mental or emotional disorders (organic brain syndrome, schizophrenia, recurrent depressive and manic-depressive disorders, and paranoid and other psychoses, plus other disorders that may become chronic) that erode or prevent the development of their func-

tional capacities in relation to three or more primary aspects of daily life—personal hygiene and self-care, self-direction, interpersonal relationships, social transactions, learning and recreation—and that erode or prevent the development of their economic self-sufficiency.

Most such individuals have required institutional care of extended duration, including intermediate-term hospitalization (90 days to 365 days in a single year), long-term hospitalization (one year or longer in the preceding five years), or nursing home placement because of a diagnosed mental condition or a diagnosis of senility without psychosis. Some such individuals have required short-term hospitalization (less than 90 days); others have received treatment from a medical or mental health professional solely on an outpatient basis, or—despite their needs—have received no treatment in the professional service system. Thus included in the target population are persons who are or were formerly residents of institutions (public and private psychiatric hospitals and nursing homes) and persons who are at high risk of institutionalization because of persistent mental disability.[5]

Counting The Chronically Mentally Ill

Since defining mental illness is difficult, it is hardly surprising that estimates of the number of people with CMI vary widely. Patients served by the mental health system are the easiest to identify and count. The number of persons outside the system is more difficult to determine. Goldman's group estimated that there were from 1.7 million to 2.4 million people with CMI in the United States out of a total of 3 million persons with severe mental disorders. These figures were derived from many sources including the 1978 report of the President's Commission on Mental Health, and data from the Bureau of the Census, the Social Security Administration, the Urban Institute, and the National Center for Social Statistics.[6]

More recent data from the NIMH Epidemiological Catchment Area Study suggests that .98 percent of the adult population has some form or combination of schizophrenia, psychosis, major affective disorder, depression, anxiety, and phobia which results in such disability that self-care is impossible.[7,8] Based on an estimated 1990 U.S. adult population of 150 million, that computes to 1.47 million persons with chronic mental illness.

Breaking down his estimate of 1.74 million people with CMI by location, Goldman determined that 900,000 were in institutions (150,000 hospitalized and 750,000 in nursing homes), and that 800,000 were in communities (690,000 in various residential settings and 110,000 who spent from 3 to 12 months of any one year in a hospital).

The current distribution of people with CMI is more difficult to gauge. Deinstitutionalization continues slowly in some states, while in others, the institutional population remains steady or even increases slightly as public sentiment questions the rationale and viability of alternative care. It is clear that were Goldman and his colleagues to rewrite their paper in 1990, they would have to include many of the homeless in a count of people with CMI.

Economic Burden Of Chronic Mental Illness

Determining the economic dimensions of chronic mental illness is difficult since the economic burden is distributed over several categories: first, the costs of care and treatment, most of which are paid for by public funds that provide services through a bewildering variety of agencies and payment mechanisms; second, income support through Social Security Income, General Relief, and other categorical benefits that vary from state to state; third, costs borne as a family burden which include out-of-pocket costs, family time spent, etc.; and fourth, loss of income due to periods of hospitalization plus pre-hospital and post-hospital time.

To illustrate the financial problems associated with chronic mental illness, we have estimated the annual costs for a seriously disabled individual. Because much of the private burden is borne by families, and much of the public burden is provided by state programs that vary in benefits, there are no precise national data to assess total costs per individual. Our best estimate, assembled from a variety of sources, uses the lowest costs possible in arriving at the figures summarized in the table below. These figures do not include medical care or costs to the criminal justice system.

CATEGORY	MEAN ANNUAL COST
Treatment, Residential, Rehabilitation Costs	16,263
Income Support (SSI, Single Person, Own Household)	4,416
Family Burden	
Dollars Spent	3,311
Time Spent @ $10 per hour	7,980
Total Yearly Cost	$31,970

Treatment, residential, and rehabilitation costs of $16,263 were estimated from the premium cost figures set by Integrated Mental Health, Inc. (IMH), a Rochester, New York, agency experimenting with capitation of services.[9] IMH enrolls individuals with major mental illnesses which are divided into three risk levels with three payment levels based on past histories of hospitalization. This figure represents an adjusted average annual cost based on numbers of patients enrolled at each level.

Income support programs, including Social Security Income (SSI), General Relief, and other support benefits, represent costs to federal and state governments for individuals unable to work or provide for themselves. The $4,416 figure is the U.S. average annual SSI support for single individuals living alone in their own households.[10] Welfare payments, a customary source of income for those not eligible for SSI, are considerably lower in most states except for Massachusetts. Single individuals on welfare living with others receive a payment of about two-thirds that of persons living on their own.

Financial demands exerted upon the families of individuals with CMI consist of out-of-pocket expenses, and the costs related to time spent on family care or arranging for care by others. The figures in the table come from a survey of 408 family members in Massachusetts who recorded the dollars spent and the time devoted to caring for a mentally ill family member.[11] Out-of-pocket expenses of $3,311 included transportation, clothing, pocket money, food, fines, damages, and legal expenses, as well as medical, psychiatric, and dental care. Time estimates included time lost from work, the number of hours spent in providing direct care, and time spent arranging for care by others. This time was valued at $10 per hour for a total of $7,980.

The total annual cost ($31,970) of illness and disability for an individual multiplied by the 1.47 million afflicted adults equals a total annual cost of caring for people with CMI in the U.S. of $46.9 billion. Of this total, $24.25 billion are treatment costs, borne chiefly by federal and state government.[12]

In addition to the cost of care and support for the most seriously mentally ill, one must also consider the social burden from loss of income that occurs when individuals become so disabled they are unable to work. Although SSI payments are intended to mitigate that loss, these payments are so low they account for only 20 percent of the average annual income of adults in this country.

Estimates of lifetime costs of illness and disability involve many factors. Among them are the expected life span of persons with CMI, ways in which changes in long-term illness require different levels of treatment, rehabilitation services, and social supports, as well as how the changes interfere with economic productivity. Data on the physical morbidity of mental illness suggest that there is a modest increase in mortality associated with these conditions, due to suicide and other causes.[13] Given our principle of caution in estimating, it seems appropriate to use age 70 as the average life span for people with CMI.

Data from longitudinal studies counter the expectation that serious mental illnesses, especially schizophrenia, are marked by inexorable deterioration.[14,15] If the later years of life are less disabling, both direct and indirect costs of the condition are correspondingly reduced. If the average age of onset of serious mental disorders is 25 and we assume that the symptoms and disabilities persist in all of those affected until an average age of 55, then treatment, residential, and rehabilitation costs must be calculated over a 30-year span. However, there is some evidence that treatment costs decrease modestly during this period. After age 55, the decline is likely to be even steeper. Harding reports that two-thirds of her elderly cohorts function "pretty well, having meaningful relationships, and most untrained observers would not think them sick."[16] Given these findings, we estimate that only one-third of those over age 55 will require treatment.

The following procedure is useful in estimating the cost of treatment over the life span. For the first five years after onset, it is assumed that treatment costs are as calculated in the table at $16,263 per year. For each five-year period after that, treatment costs are reduced by 25 percent until age 55 when treatment costs are again reduced by 25 percent and multiplied by .33 to adjust for individuals who no longer need treatment. These figures calculate to an average lifetime treatment cost of $281,695.

Total lifetime costs of mental illness can be calculated by adding lifetime treatment costs to estimates for lifetime costs of all of the other components included in the annual cost of mental illness. The same rates of decline in treatment costs, family burden, and loss of income to age 65, generate the figures in the table below. Again, these figures do not include medical care, costs to the criminal justice system, costs of various kinds of guardianship, or the capital costs of facilities.

CATEGORY	TOTAL DOLLARS
Treatment, Residential, and Rehabilitation Costs	281,695
Income Support (SSI, Single Person, Own Household)	154,339
Family Burden	
Dollars Spent	54,433
Time Spent @ $10 per hour	131,200
Total Lifetime Costs Per Person	$621,667

Figures do not discount values of future expenditures. Applying a conservative 3 percent discount, adult lifetime CMI costs would more than double.

Stigma: The Social Dimension

Persons with CMI are characteristically stigmatized by society. This affects the political response to the need for care, contributes to social isolation, and seriously interferes with the development of alternatives to institutional care. Attitudes about community housing emanate from NIMBY (Not In My Back Yard) sentiments. This attitude is experienced directly by all who work with people with CMI. By association, we share, to a greater or lesser extent, the stigma attached to our patients.

A recent study funded by The Robert Wood Johnson Foundation, The Pew Charitable Trusts, the National Institute of Mental Health, and the American Psychiatric Association sheds new light on public attitudes toward CMI. Conducted by the Yankelovich Group, the study began with focus groups to develop hypotheses. These were turned into a questionnaire administered by telephone interview to a representative sample of the U.S. population in December 1989.

The study revealed that 70 percent of Americans regard mental illness as a growing problem. Of these, 45 percent see it as a very serious health problem, although less serious than cancer, drugs, and alcoholism. Even though 40 percent have themselves experienced a mental illness or have an afflicted relative, 25 percent say they are "not at all" informed about mental illness, while another 25 percent say they are "very well" informed. While 74 percent believe that anyone can develop a mental illness and 53 percent feel that keeping up a normal life in the community will help a person with mental illness get better, less than 33 percent would welcome mental health facilities into their neighborhood. Even so, 69 percent strongly reject the idea that "the best way to handle the mentally ill is to keep them behind locked doors." Study results showed that women and young people are much more aware, concerned, tolerant, informed, and experienced about mental illness. By contrast, more affluent respondents are the least tolerant of the mentally ill.

In summary, stigma exists and is a significant factor affecting chronic mental illness. At the same time, there is an interest in knowing more and a reservoir of tolerance and understanding among people that may be brought to bear on the problem.

Notes

1. "Some Account of the Pennsylvania Hospital from its First Rise to the Beginning of the Fifth Month May, 1754," (Philadelphia: Office of the United States Gazette, 1817), 4–5.
2. DHHS Steering Committee on the CMI, "Toward a National Plan for the Chronically Mentally Ill," (December 1980), 2,17.
3. R. Manderscheid, *Personal Communication* (1990).
4. L.L. Bachrach, "Defining Chronic Mental Illness: A Concept Paper," *Hospital and Community Psychiatry* 39, No. 4 (April 1988), 383–87.
5. H.H. Goldman, A.A., Gattozzi, and C.A. Taube, "Defining and Counting the Chronically Mentally Ill," *Hospital and Community Psychiatry* 32, No. 1 (January 1981), 21–7.
6. Ibid., 24–5.

7. J.K. Myers, M.M. Weissman, G.L. Tischler, C.E. Holzer, P.J. Leaf, H. Orraschel, J.C. Anthony, J.H. Boyd, J.D. Burke, M. Kramer, and R. Stoltzman, "Six-Month Prevalence of Psychiatric Disorders in Three Communities," *Archives of General Psychiatry* 41 (1984), 959–67.

8. Department of Mental Health, Commonwealth of Massachusetts, "Prevalence Estimates for Long-term or Seriously Mentally Ill Adults," (unpublished report) (June 1989).

9. H.M. Babigian, and S.K. Reed, "A Capitated System of Care for the Seriously Mentally Ill," paper presented at the Conference on Innovation and Management of Public Mental Health Systems (Philadelphia: 1989).

10. "Background Material and Data on Programs within the Jurisdiction of the Committee on Ways and Means," U.S. House of Representatives (March 15, 1989).

11. D. Franks, "The High Cost of Caring: Economic Contribution of Families," (unpublished dissertation) (Brandeis University: 1987).

12. B. Dickey, and H.H. Goldman, "Public Health Care for the Chronically Mentally Ill," *Administration in Mental Health* 14, No. 2 (1986), 63–7.

13. J. Murphy, R.R. Monson, D.C. Olivier, A.M. Sobol, L.A. Pratt, and A.H. Leighton, "Mortality Risk and Psychiatric Disorders," *Social Psychiatry and Psychiatric Epidemiology* 24 (1989), 134–42.

14. M. Tsuang, R.F. Woolson, M.S. Fleming, "Long-Term Outcome of Psychoses," *Archives of General Psychiatry* 36 (1979), 1295–1301.

15. C.M. Harding, G.W. Brooks, T. Ashikaga, J.S. Strauss, and A. Brier, "The Vermont Longitudinal Study of Persons with Severe Mental Illness," *American Journal of Psychiatry* 144 (1987), 718–35.

16. Ibid., 722.

∽ PROBLEMS IN PROVIDING FUTURE SERVICES TO THE MENTALLY ILL

By *Herbert Pardes, MD*

In 1980, the National Institute of Mental Health (NIMH) and the Public Health Service produced a plan for the chronically mentally ill (CMI).[1] Remarkably, this concern had been partially instigated and substantially supported by a President and first lady of the United States. Presidential advisors generally counsel against such involvement since, in the battle with problems of chronic mental illness, victories are hard to win.

That national plan suggested that the Department of Health and Human Services do the following:

- Make the CMI a priority;
- Meet the service costs involved incrementally;
- Support improvement in availability and quality of care, as well as effectiveness of service in hospitals, nursing homes, and community programs;
- Develop a more effective work force to assist the CMI;
- Improve knowledge of the CMI;
- Facilitate advocacy for the CMI;
- Improve public understanding of the CMI;
- Improve collaboration among federal departments on behalf of the CMI; and
- Consider special sub-populations of the CMI.

This is a lofty and comprehensive set of recommendations. Ironically, ten years later, those recommendations with some amendments seem as pertinent as they did in 1980.

The national plan was never implemented as a whole. There have been improvements such as increased monies for research and new policies and proposals for the financing of services for the mentally ill.[2] For example, changes in federal policy have brought improved support for psychosocial rehabilitation and case management. However, some states have neither acknowledged nor implemented these changes. Many have substantial financial problems that make such changes difficult in spite of dedication to improved social and mental health services for the CMI.

Mental health professionals have worked diligently to refine psychosocial rehabilitation and related clinical services. Stein, Shore, and Gudeman[3] have been leaders in devising such mental health services. The Robert Wood Johnson Foundation has launched an impressive demonstration project, hoping to see if attractive models which integrate clear geographic authority and coordination, better housing support, and viable social and mental health services can lead to more effective programs across the country.

It is important to recognize the context in which these developments occur. Some of the most important influences on the problems of the CMI are as follows: the dramatic increase in mental health research; the extraordinary rise in citizen activism; and the government's economic conservatism and spending constraints.

Research

A close look at research in mental health and related disciplines reveals that it has never been more productive. Knowledge of the brain and its functions, biological and behavioral mechanisms and their interaction, and the role of genetics in psychiatric illness is growing at an extraordinary rate.

Epidemiological techniques for identifying and quantifying psychiatric illness have improved dramatically with some surprising results. For example, obsessive-compulsive disorders may be 50 times more common than previously identified. These new data and techniques suggest that we may be entering an era in which planning for the CMI can be more rational and systematic.

Another area of mental health research shows that genetic linkages may exist for psychiatric illnesses such as manic-depressive disease, schizophrenia, and Alzheimer's disease. Whether these linkages will be consistently replicated and whether they ultimately represent a small or large percentage of the illness population remains to be seen. The point is that genetics or other biological markers may separate subpopulations that until now had been lumped together into large categories of psychiatric disease. Such differentiation offers a number of advantages: the ability to identify selective homogeneous populations with which to do research to avoid mixing populations and nullifying effects; the potential for clearer definition of population sub-types and more informed communication which will facilitate professional collaboration among national groups and disciplines; and the development of treatment interventions and services more consistent and more tailored to the needs of a particular patient subpopulation.

Research and accumulating knowledge over several decades have contributed to increasing the number of treatments available to the mental health clinician. Twenty years ago, the problem of manic depressive disease or bipolar affective disorder was almost as formidable as that of schizophrenia today. Subsequently, the introduction of lithium and then carbamazepine modified the treatment and enhanced the functioning of many patients with bipolar disorder.

Today schizophrenia accounts for the bulk of the 1.7–2.4 million people who are considered chronically mentally ill. While medications made available over the years provided gradually increasing control, particularly over so-called "positive" symptoms such as hallucinations or delusions, the effect of chemical therapeutics on schizophrenia is still modest.

An encouraging recent development is the introduction of clozapine. According to a recent multicenter report, clozapine, after a six-week trial, lead to significant improvement in 30 percent of the schizrenics unresponsive to other medications.[4] With longer treatment time, an estimated 70 percent of "problem" or neuroleptic-refractory schizophrenics may show significant improvements in positive symptoms, negative symptoms such as isolation and apathy, and overall quality of life and functional capacity.[5] Unfortunately, in pre-approved trials in this country, clozapine was found to cause agranulocytosis in 1–2 percent of the subjects. Thus, any patient placed on clozapine will need to have blood drawn weekly to assure early detection of potentially serious side effects. This need for close monitoring in what is referred to as the Clozaril Patient Management System (CPMS) is responsible for clozapine's high cost of over $8,500 a year.

Many states must decide who should receive this medication, for how long, and what other programs will go without financial support to pay for it. For example, if someone improved only modestly on clozapine, what would determine whether the investment was worth that degree of clinical improvement? Such questions will emerge as research produces new treatments, new diagnostic tests, and new technology and services for the care of the CMI.

Another research area with thorny questions for mental health policy makers is genetics. If genetic contributions to psychiatric illnesses are documented and proven, how will this affect family planning and advice? The likelihood of a given gene being passed on to an offspring raises delicate personal and policy issues. With the help of professionals, families will have to weigh the risk that a gene will actually cause a disease in their offspring. As costly diagnostic tests are developed, cost benefit questions will also surface. In the long run, accumulated knowledge of causes and mechanisms of mental illness should be a great benefit. New treatments and service strategies should also be helpful. This rapid rush of research findings, however, means one cannot view the problems of the CMI as being fixed. Research creates a changing situation that requires flexible strategies.

In conclusion, clinical experience as well as research in therapeutics shows that a combination of biological and psychosocial therapies is often particularly effective for psychiatric patients. This was reflected in a public policy decision made recently when "medical management" was recognized by Congress as reimbursable along with other clinical treatment interventions for medical disorders. Further reexamination of related policies will be likely to stimulate other changes.

Citizen Activism

Both the numbers and the activities of citizens concerned about mental illness have grown phenomenally in the last five to ten years. The National Alliance for the Mentally Ill (NAMI), the National Depressive and Manic Depressive Association (NDMDA), the American Mental Health Fund, and the National Alliance for Research on Schizophrenia and Depression (NARSAD) were all developed in the last decade, augmenting the work of the Mental Health Association (MHA). These groups rose after the 1980 national plan was being put into final form.

Research generating increased knowledge has set in motion a favorable cycle in which patients and families more openly express concern about mental illness. The national plan called for increased advocacy and in that regard there has been some progress. Families are concerned about both the present and the future. They want the best clinical care for their ill family members now. These concerned families are also staunch advocates of research.

NAMI, MHA and NDMDA have collaborated successfully with professional groups to increase the NIMH budget; to develop a private alliance (NARSAD) for increased research support on serious psychiatric illness; and to develop state, local, and national advocacy. The American Mental Health Fund has promoted public understanding of mental illness through a national advertising campaign. Advocacy groups have also expressed concern about the quality and timeliness of provider care.

Financial Climate

These positive developments have taken place in a financial environment driven by a deficit economy. The Gramm-Rudman-Hollings law, responding to the largest financial deficits in history, epitomizes the current policy in the United States. The government has decided to constrain domestic spending rather than seek new revenues in the face of an alarming deficit and insufficient revenue.

Even before this current political trend, the Carter administration was reluctant to undertake the formidable investment demanded by the National Plan for the Chronically Mentally Ill. The Reagan administration's policy of withholding support for the services system for the mentally ill is currently being continued by the Bush administration. Indeed, the current administration is pressing for additional cuts in many related programs such as Medicare, clinical training, and federal support to local communities. The administration has also been slow to recognize the promise of mental health research; it has been Congress that substantially boosted research support in 1989 and 1990.

Since resources are scarce, policy makers have been obliged to "rob" one part of the system to "pay" other parts. Luis Marcos,[6] the mental health leader in the New York Health and Hospital Corporation, laments the concurrence of politicians and some community mental health care providers on a policy which drains the hospital system of monies and then sends these funds to providers. This leaves a system in which the community mental health care programs take care of less disabled and more motivated patients while the seriously CMI are left to languish. Marcos further decries the dismantling of the state hospital system, which he describes as the one center where such patients were given some kind of organized care. Davin Mechanic,[7] a sociologist writing on mental health policy, also noted that the functions the hospital furnished, such as housing, basic medical care, monitoring of medication compliance, etc., are not easy to provide in the community.

W. R. Shadish,[8] another writer on mental health policy, laments the primarily custodial care given in two profit-making industries that serve chronic mentally ill patients. He notes that one million such patients are cared for in nursing homes and board-and-care homes. Detailing the poor care in these privately owned facilities, he speculates that society is fundamentally disinterested in providing quality care to the chronically ill.

Aside from the contextual elements enriching, complicating, or even impeding programs for the CMI, special problems have become increasingly apparent in the last ten years. These problems somewhat modify the situation that prevailed in 1980.

First, there has been an enormous growth in the number of homeless people. An estimated one third to two-fifths of this population has significant mental impairment. Those who are both homeless and chronically mentally ill have different needs from those who may be simply homeless, for example. Those who are mentally ill have different needs from those with brain damage or alcoholism. The general problem of homelessness has attracted the attention of society, and there have been some attempts to address it. However, at least one important underlying cause of homelessness, chronic mental illness, has not received adequate attention. It may well be that if the issue of homelessness does stir the general American public, it can lead to a greater awareness and sensitivity to the needs of the CMI.

A second special problem is the mentally ill patient who is also chemically abusive. There are now many more such patients. N. L. Cohen, another student of mental health policy, and Marcos[9] have reported that the use of alcohol and drugs in the psychiatric setting, as well as the crack epidemic, have made patients far more violent according to hospital staffs. These dual-diagnosis patients are often neglected because of poorly organized services and the formidable care required.

In 1985, John Talbott, who has given special attention to the chronically mentally ill in his career, noted a third development.[10] A large number of young chronic patients, many never before hospitalized, became as dysfunctional as long-term patients in state hospitals. Leona Bachrach,[11] a widely regarded mental health policy authority, cites this as evidence that lengthy institutionalization alone is not necessarily the cause of chronicity.

The young chronics pose a special problem. They use psychiatric services in a hit-or-miss manner, shifting from one facility to another. Often they become involved with the criminal justice system as well. They cannot form stable relationships and their support systems are almost nonexistent. This subgroup of the CMI presents a unique and formidable challenge for clinical care givers and care takers.

Suggestions For Action

The problems of the CMI are imposing. Finances, housing, food, medication, psychosocial rehabilitation, and coordination of services must be considered. Good providers must be selected and trained. Caretakers and clinical care givers must be motivated, sustained, and given adequate respite. The CMI must have opportunities to do useful and productive work, and opportunities to make and sustain relationships. All of these points and more have to be considered in order to meet the full challenge.

It is impossible to formulate any easy or global answers to the problems of the CMI. However, the following suggestions can provide a beginning. First, it may be time for another Presidential or Congressional commission whose goal is not just fiscal solutions for problems of mental health services for the CMI. Rather the goal can be to define the steps needed to correct the entire problem and prioritize those steps. This is a population, however, whose vital service needs are many and prioritizing one service need above another will inevitably deny some patients vital services. It seems hopeless to anticipate any national readiness to provide the kinds of resources that the comprehensive 1980 plan suggested. Still, the nation's conscience regarding homelessness has been stirred and attention can be directed at the mentally ill homeless which constitutes a substantial portion of the homeless population.

The Robert Wood Johnson Foundation (RWJF) experiment is important in this regard. It should be determined if the RWJF program has sufficiently altered the plan of any one city for it to serve as a model. Perhaps with the help of a special federal demonstration project along with foundation or private support, such a model could be more broadly disseminated and tested around the country.

On the other hand, what may be critical is whether at the federal or state level we can delineate a plan that unfolds in stages. This would be more fiscally realistic but also more challenging. Perhaps key parts of a comprehensive plan could be selected for focus, such as the responsibility for housing or total mental health services for a defined group.

Second, related health care developments may influence the mental health situation. Leona Bachrach[12] has pointed out that because health care is available to all in some nations in Western Europe, these countries take a somewhat different stance on care of the CMI. For example, in the United Kingdom, where there is universal access, it is only a matter of time before the patient is admitted to service. There has been some political interest in covering currently uninsured citizens with health care in the United States. A new national commission or plan could articulate the rationale that the CMI be included in any plan to provide wider access to health care and that other health and social policy be carefully reviewed for potential impact on the CMI.

Third, progress made in the development of citizen groups is laudatory. The NIMH Director has created a national mental health forum to bring together various professional and citizen groups. Perhaps it is appropriate for foundations to help these groups focus on advocacy on behalf of the CMI. The citizen groups might mount a plan of private investment for the CMI if the government cannot provide it, or complement an existing government effort.

Fourth, any set of options must involve substantial support for research. The basic causes of schizophrenia and other serious mental illnesses, the development of better therapeutics, the investigation of the service system to see what programs work and for which patients, and programs tailored to fit the multiple subgroups referred to earlier are all proper themes for such research. Research on mental illness in this country was stymied between the mid-sixties and mid-seventies but has blossomed over the last dozen years. There is much catching up to be done. The training of young researchers, the support of senior researchers, and funding for the necessary clinical settings and capital facilities to conduct such research are all critical.

In addition, research on the nature of chronicity and the clinical course of such illnesses is important. Dr. Fran Cournos, chief of the Washington Heights Mental Health Service in New York City, proposes that patients be considered at risk for chronic psychiatric illness at the time of the first episode. Dr. Cournos suggests further that researchers focus on which patients stay in treatment, which use drugs and alcohol, and which factors contribute to chronicity. Concurrently, health care professionals must help caretakers sustain the motivation and resulting gratification enabling them to care for people with CMI in a continuously supportive and sensitive fashion. A follow-up research program on patient compliance would also be most valuable.

Eventually, research should also clarify information about the various subpopulations of the CMI. For instance, how does a family subgroup with an eye tracking defect compare to another with a linkage to chromosome 5, or still another subgroup with enlarged ventricles of the brain? Are different treatments necessary? Are different residential and social supports necessary for these various populations?

Fifth, it would be advantageous to have a national commission solely on housing the mentally ill. A paucity of subsidized living facilities throughout the country, along with the loss of single-room dwellings in large cities, has much to do with the enormous population of people on the streets. While rushing to deinstitutionalize and to shift patients from one clinical treatment setting to another, many policy makers forgot that these people must have a place to live, food to eat, and money with which to support themselves. It might be appropriate to place emphasis on improving one service, such as housing, while other services remain constant as a reference standard. Thus the relative importance of each service could be systematically determined.

Sixth, care givers who take total responsibility for the CMI in their charge could be reimbursed for their participation in demonstration projects in clinical mental health delivery. Surprisingly, in some settings, a multidisciplinary team taking on a certain number of CMI can provide reasonably good services that are sustained and continuous. The NIMH conducted demonstration projects which led to the widespread use of case managers and community support programs. Community support, medication, social skills training, and attention to the family's needs and issues are interventions that seem to reduce hospitalization and to contribute to better functioning of the CMI. Consolidating various helpful interventions into demonstration projects might be advisable in testing a more comprehensive model.

Seventh, in all of these deliberations, the heterogeneity of the individuals with chronic mental illness must be kept uppermost in mind. The young chronic differs from the long institutionalized middle-aged individual. The person afflicted with schizophrenia who also has used crack or alcohol has a different set of problems than the schizophrenic who has not. Patients in large cities have much more fragmented family and social support systems than the CMI in less heavily populated communities, and this has to be taken into account. Any strategy not attentive to these differences will be inadequate. Perhaps a demonstration may be attempted with specific subpopulations along these lines.

Deciding what to do next with broad approaches, rather than individual technical correction and tinkering, constitutes a formidable challenge. Vigorous advocacy of priority for the CMI is crucial. However, the direction chosen may be strongly determined by the realities. The development of a national plan for the CMI was laudatory. However, it suggested that an enormous amount could be done when in all likelihood that was never true. It did lay out a game plan. Some of that game plan has not changed, but the special problems of the last decade will need to be accounted for in any future plan.

To effect a large change, one either has to have substantial political clout or one has to demonstrate a model sufficiently attractive to induce others to replicate it. Or one can develop a program in measured increments by putting a working system into place.

The good news is that treatments have improved somewhat; the bad news is that they still have a long way to go. The research is exciting with great potential, but we must be careful not to raise expectations too high. Practical outcome from research takes time. Citizen and professional groups form the framework from which a very substantial advocacy group could be marshalled. These identified citizen, consumer, and professional groups probably number in excess of a million individuals and might reach tens of millions if the advocacy effort really snowballed.

Many would say that a society is measured by how it responds to those who are most needy. This country has hardly been exemplary in that regard; unfortunately few countries can boast better track records. The problem is formidable, complex, and costly, but it is no less critical today than it was in 1980.

Notes

1. "Toward a National Plan for the Chronically Mentally Ill," from a report to the Secretary by the Department of Health and Human Services Steering

Committee on the Chronically Mentally Ill, (December, 1980).

2. R.G. Frank and H.H. Goldman, "Financing Care of the Severely Mentally Ill: Incentives, Contracts, and Public Responsibility," *Journal of Social Issues* 45, No. 3, (1989), 131–44.

3. M.F. Shore and J.E. Gudeman, "Seeing the Chronically Mentally Ill in an Urban Setting," *New Directions for Mental Health Services* 39 (Fall 1988).

4. J. Kane, G. Honigfeld, J. Singer, and H. Melter, "Clozapine for the Treatment-Resistant Schizophrenic: A Double-Blind Comparison with Chlorpromazine," *Archives of General Psychiatry* 45, No. 9 (1988), 789–96.

5. Ibid., 789–96.

6. L. Marcos, "Who Profits from Deinstitutionalization?" *Hospital and Community Psychiatry* 40, No. 2 (December 1989), 1221.

7. D. Mechanic, "Strategies for Improved Care of the Seriously Mentally Ill," *Milbank Quarterly* 65, No. 2, (1987), 203–30.

8. W.R. Shadish, Jr., "Private-Sector Care for Chronically Mentally Ill Individuals: The More Things Change, the More They Stay the Same," *American Psychologist* 44, No. 8 (August 1989), 1142–7.

9. N.L. Cohen and L.R. Marcos, "The Bad-Mad Dilemma for Public Psychiatry," *Hospital and Community Psychiatry* 40, No. 7 (July 1989), 677.

10. J.A. Talbott, "Commentary: The Emerging Crisis in Chronic Care," *The Young Adult Chronic Patient, Collected Articles from Hospital and Community Psychiatry* (1981), 1.

11. L.L. Bachrach, "Young Adult Chronic Patients: An Analytic Review of the Literature," *The Young Adult Chronic Patient, Collected Articles from Hospital and Community Psychiatry* (1982), 2–10.

12. L.L. Bachrach, "The Chronic Patient, Some Reflections from Abroad," *Hospital and Community Psychiatry* 40, No. 6 (June 1989), 573–4.

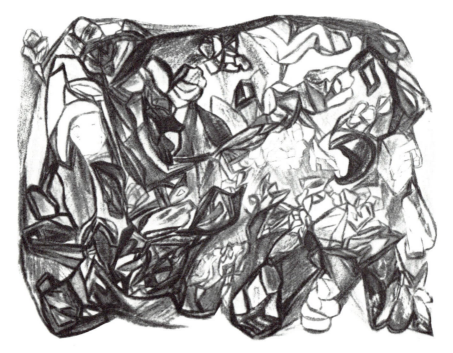

Abstract Composition by an "Inmate" of an Insane Asylum. Discovered by Hans Prinzhorn, MD; Courtesy of The Bettmann Archive.

∽ FILLING THE GAPS
Service Gaps and Exemplary Programs in the
Treatment of Chronic Mentally Ill Persons

By Leonard I. Stein, MD

To date, we neither know how to cure nor prevent chronic mental illness. However, over the past 20 years we have learned much about how to improve its management. It is an illness plagued by remissions and relapse into psychosis. In most cases, we can effectively treat the psychotic phase of the illness with medication combined with a supportive environment. Frequently, hospitalization is also necessary. During a quiescent period, the patient is generally in touch with reality, but does suffer from other impairments which interfere with his/her ability to make an unassisted stable adjustment to community life. Typical impairments are as follows: sensitivity to stress, difficulty with interpersonal relationships, a deficit in coping skills, and difficulty in transferring learning from one site to another. These impairments are secondary to one or a combination of the negative symptoms of schizophrenia, personality disorder, a residual psychotic process, or organicity. In order to understand the current problems in treating persons with chronic mental illness (CMI), it is useful to address some of the service gaps in the treatment of these two phases of chronic mental illness, as well as to describe some exemplary service models of care and treatment. First, it is necessary to explain the typical course of treatment for chronic mentally ill persons.

Therapeutic strategy for chronic mental illness must address both the psychotic and long-term impairment phases with a double-pronged approach. The first is primarily medical and is aimed at interrupting the psychotic phase as rapidly as possible. The long-term impairment phase requires a more rehabilitative focus designed to increase functional capacity and psychological stability through skill training, psychological and environmental supports, and, when indicated, maintenance medication. The thrust of both prongs increases stability and functional capacity to a greater degree than either one could do alone.

The major clinical problem in treating persons with chronic mental illness is helping them to make a stable adjustment to community life. They need what the rest of us do—a place to live; an opportunity to socialize; useful vocational or avocational activities that anchor the day and give meaning to life; financial independence; medical services; mental health services; and, at times, crisis resolution services. The only need persons with CMI have that the rest of us do not is professional support within the community in which they live. Indeed, any organization that works with this population must support the community in learning how to relate to the mentally ill that are a part of that community. This is just as important as providing direct support to these patients.

In describing the range of services provided for the person with CMI, it is useful to organize the field into three domains—specific interventions, programs, and systems.

Specific interventions are tightly defined and narrowly focused treatments for a specific disorder. They can range from a medication, such as lithium for the treatment of mania, to psychoeducational work with a family that has a member with schizophrenia. Programs typically unite a group of mental health professionals to meet a given service need. The program may provide one or more specific interventions. Examples range from an outpatient crisis intervention service to an inpatient ward. Ultimately a system of care is comprised of specific interventions and programs that function together to provide coordinated and comprehensive services.

In devising systems of care for treatment of persons with CMI, it is critical to fill the service gaps that exist in the field. Exemplary services are innovative attempts to solve problems which are centered around the two phases of chronic mental illness—the psychotic phase and the long-term impairment phase. Exemplary services are further organized along the domains of the specific interventions, programs, and systems.

Psychotic Phase And Treatment

In most cases, we can effectively treat the psychotic phase of the illness; however, an estimated 10 to 20 percent of patients do not respond to neuroleptic treatment.[1] Until very recently, we have had no new breakthroughs in effective medication for the psychotic phases of schizophrenia, manic illness, or depressive illness. The anti-psychotics, the anti-depressants, and lithium came on the scene many years ago. These produce significant side effects, especially the anti-psychotics, with extrapyramidal symptoms and tardive dyskinesia.

A new medication called Clozapine is the first anti-psychotic medication in the past quarter century whose pharmacologic characteristics significantly differ from earlier anti-psychotic drugs.[2] It has eliminated psychotic symptoms in a significant percentage of patients unresponsive to earlier drugs. It does not carry with it the uncomfortable extrapyramidal symptoms or disfiguring problems of tardive dyskinesia. However, it does present the risk of causing agranulocytosis in approximately 1–2 percent of those treated. In addition to helping patients with refractory positive symptoms, it has also been reported to have some amelioratory effect on negative symptoms. Clozapine also has major potential for opening the door to a whole new class of medications that may not carry the hematopoetic suppression properties typical of Clozapine itself.

A major gap in our services to persons with chronic mental illness is in the continuum of response to persons experiencing psychotic symptoms. Although psychotic symptoms vary from early emergence of paranoia experienced as suspiciousness to full-blown psychosis, the response available in many communities consists of outpatient treatment or treatment in a psychiatric hospital with no services in between. Although many communities have crisis intervention services, they typically operate as evaluation or disposition units that make one assessment and then refer patients elsewhere for treatment. These services are commonly located in hospital emergency rooms, often serving as little more than a conduit to hospital psychiatric wards. The typical mental health crisis service is neither conceptualized nor structured to be actively involved in resolving crisis situations and stabilizing patients. Crisis units that function this way do little to meet the varying needs of patients during a relapse period.

There are several good examples of exemplary services that fill the gaps in service to psychiatric patients. One exemplary crisis service can be found in Dane County, Wisconsin.[3] This service provides 24-hour, 7-day-a-week crisis resolution using a mobile team to assist persons in crisis. A 24-hour telephone response unit works closely with the mobile team. The mobile crisis team and the crisis phone unit form an integrated crisis service. Unlike the evaluation and disposition units described above, this unit is charged with responsibility for resolving the crisis. This may require multiple daily contact over several weeks, and will often require the involvement of family and social service agencies, as well as community members from landlords to neighbors. A crisis unit like the one in Dane County can also help to fill the major gaps between a patient's home and the hospital. An integrated crisis service also offers other alternatives. The patient's residence becomes viable when mental health professionals can actually go to the home to provide support to the patient and the patient's family. If remaining with the family during the period of crisis is too stressful, the patient can spend the night in a hotel and the unit team can monitor the patient during daytime hours as well. When that is not sufficient, a crisis bed can be provided.

The crisis bed model is another exemplary service that was developed by the Southwest Denver Community Health Center in the early 1970s.[4] Families with one or two spare bedrooms take a crisis patient into their homes and provide room, board, and client care for a modest fee. The family is provided a great deal of consultation and support by a mobile crisis team that is available 24 hours a day, 7 days a week. The patients participate in family chores and activities, and meaningful personal relationships often develop between family sponsors and patients. Attention is paid to matching patients with families. This model was carefully researched by the Southwest Denver Group, which found that the vast majority of patients who would ordinarily be hospitalized could be managed very well in the crisis bed model. A growing number of communities in the United States now use this exemplary service.

A third alternative between home and the hospital ward is the Inn program developed at the Massachusetts Mental Health Center.[5] A small locked psychiatric unit providing a high degree of supervision and nursing care is integrated with a considerably less supervised living situation termed the Inn. The Inn operates as a day hospital, providing a variety of therapeutic activities. The Inn also offers transitional residence for patients who currently have no other place to live. The boundary between the Inn and the locked unit is permeable so that the bureaucratic barriers are markedly reduced. Thus, persons who require a high degree of supervision can receive it when they need it. When less supervision is required, they can easily move back to the Inn. This mode is not only economically efficient, but clinically sensible.

Long-Term Impairment Phase And Treatment

There is a paucity of services that help patients reduce their relapse rate and make a stable and satisfying life in the community. Because of their long-term impairments, patients have difficulty maintaining the necessities required for stability, such as housing, finances, socialization, and meaningful work or daily activities. Absence of these necessities leads to patient stress which may cause relapse. Currently patients with chronic mental illness in the United States experience a 60 percent relapse rate in the year following discharge from a hospital. This disruption significantly reduces their quality of life.

The following four exemplary services address this service gap: the Assertive Mobile Community Treatment team that focuses on a population generally resistant to services, thus requiring a great deal of outreach; the Club model, which serves patients who are more willing to come in and participate in the program; the Lodge model, which combines communal living with work; and psychoeducational interventions with families.

The Assertive Mobile Community Treatment (AMCT) team program is designed to work with the most difficult-to-treat patients in the system.[6] This program is also referred to as the Training in Community Living (TCL) program, and the Program for Assertive Community Treatment (PACT). The patients targeted by this program often resist coming in regularly for services so they need assertive outreach. They often are not compliant with medications; need some daily structure in their lives; are poor at monitoring their illness—often interpreting symptoms as being externally caused; tend to have frequent and severe crises; and have a tenuous social network. Prior to being involved with the AMCT team, they had frequent relapses with repeated hospitalizations. The AMCT program was developed to help persons with CMI live in the community, decrease their need for psychiatric hospitalizations, and enhance their quality of life. Much of the program provides help with daily living; teaches patients coping skills so that over time they can accomplish things on their own; and provides a support system for patients who have little social support or human contact. Much of the treatment involves practical activities such as helping a patient maintain his or her apartment, shop for groceries, or use a washing machine at a local laundromat. Verbal interaction between staff and patients is important. However, it is easier for many of these patients to relate to those who are helping them meet concrete needs than talk with a therapist in an office. Two key parts of the program are assertive outreach and strong case management. The latter assures that patients' needs are being met, that problems are recognized early in their development, and that patients do not drop out of treatment. This model was carefully researched, and that research has been replicated several times with the consistent finding of reduction in hospitalization and increased patient functioning.[7]

The second exemplary service developed to fill service gaps for more stable patients is the Clubhouse model. This was pioneered by Fountain House in New York City.[8] The program has a vocational emphasis providing basic skill training, social support, and a meaningful way to structure time. People with CMI who attend the Clubhouse are considered "members," and the program is arranged so that it cannot function without the services the members provide. Members answer telephones, cook meals, and take care of minor maintenance. Even some of the outreach services to members who have not been attending are provided by other members. Professional staff supply structure and supervision, but once the culture is established, even much of this responsibility falls to the members. The hallmark of this program is its optimistic view of each patient's potential to grow into a fully functioning member of society. As is clear from the description, the usual situation of patients being dependent on staff is discouraged. Instead, interdependence among patients is strongly encouraged. The term "empowerment" has been used to describe this process. This model is now operating in approximately 200 communities across the nation.

The Lodge program developed by George Fairweather is another exemplary program that helps people enjoy a sustained and meaningful community life. A group of patients in a long-term ward live and work together as a group in the hospital. They are then moved en masse into a community residence. The patients support each other in the living situation, and they also work together as a cottage industry, providing something practical, such as a janitorial service or painting service to the community. The hospital staff continue to be involved with the group in the community, but gradually wean themselves away. Like the Clubhouse model, the Lodge has had many replications and is operating with scores of programs throughout the country.

This past decade has seen renewed interest in working with families that have a member with schizophrenia. The psychoeducational approach differs markedly from previous ones, both in theory and application. Formerly, family therapy was based on the assumption that family pathology was a major cause of schizophrenia. Interventions were developed to identify the pathology and attempt to deal with it. Parents of children with schizophrenia became angry because they felt that their therapists were blaming them for the illness and were treating them with hostility. In addition, there is no substantial evidence that these approaches were doing any good. Psychoeducational intervention is very different. It assumes that schizophrenia is an illness with a strong biological component. It views the family and the patient as both being victims of the disease and searches to identify misconceptions and problems with which patients and their families are having difficulty. The approach is to educate about the illness and to help patients and their families learn problem-solving strategies. Several studies have now demonstrated a marked reduction in relapse rates in families being treated with this approach.[9]

A second monumental problem for persons with CMI is the shortage of decent and affordable community housing. While this need is most evident with the burgeoning numbers of homeless mentally ill, it also applies to the tens of thousands of other persons with CMI now living in substandard board-and-care homes. Providing housing in and of itself is not sufficient; most persons with chronic mental illness need support in their housing in order to make it in the community over the long term. It is now recognized that persons with chronic mental illness can live much more independently than was thought possible if they are provided with a visiting staff that can help with daily activities, such as cleaning, meal preparation, laundry, and money management.

Two exemplary programs dealing with community housing have already been mentioned—the Assertive Mobile Community Treatment team and the Clubhouse. These programs help in several ways. Two or three compatible patients can be brought together to share an apartment they couldn't possibly afford on their own. Or the agency serving the clients can become the renter, sign the lease, pay the security deposit, pay the rent to the landlord, and then collect the rent from the patients. This is a tremendous help for many patients who cannot provide the security deposit and first month's rent for an apartment. After a year or two, the agency can recoup its initial expenditure and have the patients sign the lease independently. In addition, the AMCT team will visit the patient in the home frequently to provide the helpful support services described earlier.

A third major gap in helping the person with CMI live a quality life in the community is the lack of meaningful work available to them. Most people with CMI are unable to work in competitive employment 8 hours a day, 5 days a week. Research has shown that even with adequate training and assistance in finding work, the person with CMI has difficulty sustaining employment. For instance, Thresholds, a psychosocial rehabilitation agency in Chicago, was extremely successful in finding jobs for persons with CMI but reported that six months later, less than 37 percent were still working.[10]

Nevertheless, two exemplary programs, one pioneered by Fountain House and the other by Thresholds, show great promise. The model developed by Fountain House is called Transitional Employment Program (TEP).[11] Here, a job with a typically high turnover rate is located in the competitive market. Fountain House approaches the employer to fill that job. The job is to be filled by the organization and not by an individual. Fountain House will then enlist three or four of its members to do that job, providing a staff worker to train and supervise the members on the job. Thus, members are involved in actual competitive employment, gain work experience, supplement their disability checks with needed income, improve their self-esteem, and hopefully move on to permanent employment. The TEP placements last for 6 months, at which time members are rotated either to permanent jobs or to other TEP sites. If a member does not show up for work, the staff person will take over that responsibility to ensure that the work is done. The employer has the satisfaction of reducing job turnover, and the TEP members benefit greatly.

The second program is the supported work model developed by Thresholds. It is similar to the the supported housing model, postulating that people with CMI can work permanently in competitive settings provided they are given ongoing support.[12] That support is provided by a staff person who has established a relationship with both the client and the employer and is available for assistance at any time. The intervention varies flexibly from intensive support over a short time to infrequent and brief supportive visits. The essential element is close monitoring to determine how much intervention is needed. Early results of an experiment on this model being done by Thresholds show that an encouraging percentage of patients can remain competitively employed.

These exemplary models aim to help patients live more independent lives than they have in the past. However, many patients still feel too dependent on the treatment system and find their sense of self-esteem eroded by this dependency. The self-help movement is directed towards reducing patients' dependency on the service system and increasing interdependency among patients, thereby increasing a sense of independence, competence, and self-esteem.[13] These consumer-operated services (a term preferred over patient self-help groups) provide three primary services: crisis phone lines, drop-in centers, and safe-houses. Crisis phone lines provide telephone support in times of stress. Drop-in centers offer places for socialization and mutual support, and safe-houses are locations where people can come and stay from a day to several days to gain safety and support. All of these measures are staffed by the consumers of the services.

Service Failings

Two areas of need are so important and so deficient that they may more appropriately be called failings than gaps. The first is a failure to educate. Professional schools are not providing multi-disciplinary training to their students who will be caring for persons with CMI. As noted earlier, over the past 20 years, there has been an explosion in our knowledge of the services required to treat the chronically disabled psychiatric patient. The accepted way of providing those services is through a multi-disciplinary core team of psychiatrists, nurses, and social workers with the addition of rehabilitation counselors, occupational therapists, and other specialists. Currently, training in this new technology is primarily through postgraduate continuing education courses; symposia at meetings of various professional associations; workshops by the community support program branch of the NIMH; and a host of state and regional workshops and conferences on the chronic patient. These training sessions ordinarily focus on the conceptual and day-to-day care of the individual with CMI. Although they mention the multi-disciplinary composition of the team, they rarely address multi-disciplinary collaboration. There is literally a handful of programs in the country exposing trainees to the psychosocial treatment of persons with CMI in the community, and there is a virtual absence of interdisciplinary training. As a result, the majority of professionals graduating from these training programs is ill-equipped to play a full role in community treatment programs.

The second and even larger problem is the failure to provide a system of care for those who suffer from chronic mental illness. Most communities cannot appropriately address the clinical problems of our patients because they do not have comprehensive and integrated services. A brief historical overview of the development of mental health services in the United States will help explain the roots of this organizational problem.

In the middle 1800s, Dorothea Dix, concerned about the neglect of the mentally ill, lobbied states to take on the responsibility for their care. The states responded by building hospitals to house and treat the mentally ill. In addition, over the past three decades, a variety of community services were developed to treat this population. These services were developed at different times, funded by different sources, and have different philosophies and priorities. In virtually every state, the hospital and community programs neither coordinate nor collaborate, often competing for funds and transferring patients from their care to other programs that are equally unequipped to take responsibility. Together these services comprise a "non-system" of mental health care in which a few patients get more than they need, many patients get less than they need, and some get nothing at all. Patients commonly get lost in this non-system, with no one feeling obligated to seek them out. When patients refuse to follow a program's rules, they typically are terminated from the program by staff who believe there is no other choice. Patients are moved from the community into the hospital, and from the hospital back into the community to the extent that the hospital, the community, the patient, and the family all feel mistreated. This non-system is failing the patient and undermining the potential effectiveness of the professionals working in it.

To move from a non-system to a system of care requires fundamental changes in funding mental health services, including decentralized control of the planning, organizing, and financing of services. It also involves changing the fundamental strategy of working with this population from the failed time-limited approach to a rehabilitative one that focuses on supporting and helping patients grow while achieving sustained tenure in the community. In a system of care, hospital and community programs do not compete with each other, but see each other as providing complementary services to patients during different phases of their illness.

In all of this fragmentation of services to the individuals with CMI, there have been two exemplary systems of care. The first is the effort that was started in Dane County, Wisconsin, in the mid-1970s.[14] The Dane County system has now become sufficiently developed to provide a training ground for others who wish to follow its excellent example. The other exemplary effort is one that was spearheaded by The Robert Wood Johnson Foundation in its national initiative, the

Program On Chronic Mental Illness.[15] That program has focused on helping nine of our largest cities evolve from non-systems to systems of care. This program has attracted national attention, and some of those cities are doing exceptionally well. This success has encouraged other states and cities to emulate their practices.

In conclusion, the problems and gaps noted earlier—lack of safe medication for the psychotic episode of mental illness; a poor continuum of alternatives to acute hospitalization; insufficient programs to help patients make a sustained and decent life in the community; the shortage in housing; the shortage of work opportunities; the shortage of consumer-operated services; inadequate professional training; and fragmented non-systems of care—are the rule rather than the exception. The exemplary services developed to fill these gaps have not been widely disseminated and are too scarce to help the hundreds of thousands of people with CMI who need them. These exemplary services are like isolated beacons of light in the darkness, reminding us that we know how to do much more than we are doing. Perhaps the greatest problem of all is our failure to widely implement these exemplary programs.

Notes

1. J. Kane, G. Honigfeld, J. Singer, and H. Meltzer, "Clozapine for the Treatment-Resistant Schizophrenic," *Archives of General Psychiatry*, 45, No. 9 (1988), 789–96.
2. Ibid., 789–96
3. L.I. Stein, R.J. Diamond, and R.M. Factor, "A System Approach to the Care of Persons with Schizophrenia," eds. M.I. Herz, S.J. Keith, J.P. Docherty, *Handbook of Schizophrenia*, 5 (Amsterdam: Elsevier Science Publishers, 1990).
4. R.R. Polak, M.W. Kirby, and W.S. Deitchman, "Treating Acutely Psychotic Patients in Private Homes," ed. H.R. Lamb, *New Directions for Mental Health Services*, 1 (San Francisco: Jossey-Bass, 1979), 49–64.
5. J. Gudeman, M. Shore, and B. Dickey, "Day Hospitalization at an Inn instead of Inpatient Care for Psychiatric Patients," ed. M.F. Shore, J.E. Gudeman, *New England Journal of Medicine*, 308 (San Francisco: Jossey-Bass, 1983), 749–53.
6. L.I. Stein, and M.A. Test, "An Alternative to Mental Hospital Treatment: Conceptual Model, Treatment Program, and Clinical Evaluation," *Archives of General Psychiatry* 37 (1980), 392–97.
7. L.I. Stein, "Funding a System of Care for Schizophrenia," *Psychiatric Annals* 17 (1987), 592–98.
8. J.H. Beard, R.N. Propst, and T.J. Malamud, "The Fountain House Model of Psychiatric Rehabilitation," *Psychosocial Rehabilitation Journal* V (1982), 47–53.
9. M.J. Goldstein, "New Developments in Interventions with Families of Schizophrenics," *New Directions for Mental Health Services* (special issue 1981), 12.

10. Thresholds' proposal to The Robert Wood Johnson Foundation's Mental Health Services Development Program (1987).

11. Beard, 47–53.

12. Staff, "Supported Employment for Psychiatrically Disabled Adults," *Community Support Network News*, 3 {special issue} (April 1987), 4.

13. R.W. Glover, and S. Steber "From the Back Wards to the Boardroom: The Empowerment of Mental Health Consumers," (1989) paper presented at a University of Pennsylvania conference entitled "Innovation and Management in Public Health Systems," Philadelphia, Pennsylvania.

14. L.I. Stein and L.J. Ganser, "System for Funding Mental Health Services," in ed. J.A. Talbott, *New Directions for Mental Health*, 18 (San Francisco: Jossey-Bass, 1983), 25–32.

15. L.H. Aiken, S.A. Somers, and M.F. Shore, "Private Foundations in Health Affairs: A Case Study of the Development of a National Initiative for the Chronically Mentally Ill," *American Psychologist*, 41 (1986), 1290–95.

~ ORGANIZING AND FINANCING CARE FOR THE CHRONICALLY MENTALLY ILL IN THE UNITED STATES

By Howard H. Goldman, MD, PhD, and Richard G. Frank, PhD

History

Almost from the beginning, financing policy has shaped the organization of care for the chronically mentally ill (CMI) in the United States. Increasing indigence in the early 19th century created a shift of care from private institutions to newly-created public institutions. States built and staffed public asylums, but local governments were responsible for payment of care. Many communities decided to house the CMI locally in almshouses and jails to avoid the higher cost of care in state asylums. By the turn of the 20th century, however, social reformers argued that care of the mentally ill should be a state responsibility rather than a local one. A series of state care acts centralized care and financing of the mentally ill in state-operated and state-financed asylums. As local communities shifted the burden of responsibility onto the state, senility was reclassified a mental illness, and the indigent elderly were sent along with the CMI to state institutions.[1]

The federal government created a National Asylum in Washington D.C., but otherwise played a minor role in the care of the CMI until after World War II. The federal Community Mental Health legislation of the 1960s initiated development of mental health centers in communities throughout the United States. These were predicated on the concept that early treatment in local communities would prevent chronicity and shrink the populations in state mental hospitals. At the same time, the Medicare and Medicaid amendments to the federal Social Security Act provided insurance benefits to the elderly, poor, and disabled, including the CMI. Federal policymakers, however, limited the mental health benefits in Medicare and Medicaid to restrict the shifting of costs from states to the federal government and preserve the historic role of state care. Although limited, the benefits did enable states to share the cost of care for the CMI with the federal government.

Unfortunately, community mental health centers did not adequately address the needs of the CMI. Responding to this problem, the National Institute of Mental Health encouraged many states to develop community support programs for the CMI. The Mental Health Systems Act of 1980 was intended to greatly expand federal resources for the Community Support Program. In 1981, most of this legislation was repealed with the change in administration. As a result, the growth in federal financing was stopped.[2]

State governments remain the dominant payer for the CMI, followed by the federal government, along with a much smaller contribution from local government sources. Although local governments pay for as much as 50 percent of the costs of ambulatory services for the CMI in some communities, they rarely support more than 10 percent of the total cost of care, including hospital services. State government plays a much greater role in care for mental illness than for general medical care, while the federal role is correspondingly smaller. Overall, financing has been complex and restricted; no one has wanted to pay. The result has been a highly differentiated and decentralized system of discontinuous care in which the CMI often have been neglected and abandoned, whether they were treated in institutions or in their communities.[3]

Current System of Services

The current system of mental health services follows the contour of the financial systems that support it. There is a complex two-class system of care divided between public and private sectors. There are public and private institutions and agencies, and there are public and private payers. Occasionally, private resources are used to pay for care in a public institution; for example, private insurance may cover the care of an individual committed to a state mental hospital. More commonly, public resources, such as Medicare or Medicaid, are used to pay for care in a private agency.

The system of care is also divided between institutional and non-institutional sectors. Hospitals and nursing homes provide institutional services to approximately a million of the CMI each year. Hospital services are provided in public and private free-standing psychiatric hospitals; in psychiatric units, in public and private general hospitals, and community mental health centers; and in general medical and surgical beds in community hospitals. Non-institutional services are provided to about a million of the CMI living in communities in an even wider array of public and private settings. These include clinics, psychosocial rehabilitation programs, providers' offices, and day and night hospitals.[4]

Out-of-pocket expenses account for a small proportion of the care of the CMI, usually occurring during the early stages of illness before it has become disabling. Governmental resources finance care directly through public facilities or through a variety of ways to contract with private providers. Third-party mechanisms include private insurance and public payers, such as Medicare and Medicaid.

When insured individuals first develop mental illness, private resources are used to pay for care, usually in physicians' offices, hospitals, and clinics. As the illness progresses, individuals often incur huge expenses. Typically, the co-payments for the treatment of mental illness are higher than for general medical illness, and often there are limits on insurance coverage. If insurance is tied to employment, such benefits are lost when a mentally ill person becomes disabled. After having spent substantial sums, even while covered by insurance, such an individual usually becomes uninsurable. If he or she is eligible for Social Security Disability Insurance (SSDI) benefits, the individual also becomes eligible for Medicare, but only after two years on SSDI. If a person becomes destitute in the interim, however, he or she may be covered by Medicaid.

Medicare, a federal program supported through payroll deductions and voluntary premiums, covers the acute care of elderly and disabled former workers. It covers inpatient care in a general hospital but only a lifetime total of 190 days of inpatient care in a free-standing psychiatric hospital. Until 1987, only $500 in outpatient treatment costs were reimbursed with a 50 percent patient co-payment, meaning that Medicare only paid $250 per year as a maximum. Legislation in 1987 raised the limit in two steps to $2,200 ($1,100 in Medicare payment). Legislation in 1989 eliminated the ceiling entirely. Brief office visits for medical management of psychotropic drugs have been exempted from the limit since 1987, when the special co-payment schedule was also dropped.[5] This change directly benefits the CMI Medicare beneficiary by removing barriers to appropriate treatment. Prior to the 1987 legislation, partial hospital care was reimbursed only in hospital-based programs, and services such as homecare, case management, and rehabilitation have not been reimbursed. The 1987 statute called for regulations to redefine the partial hospital benefit. Although Medicare is primarily a program for the elderly (90 percent of all expenditures are spent on the corresponding 90 percent of beneficiaries over the age of 65 years), one-half of all Medicare mental health expenditures are incurred by the non-elderly who qualify because of disability.[6]

Medicaid, a federal–state partnership financed through general revenues, is a much more flexible program offering a diversity of hospital and non-hospital acute and long-term care services to the CMI. Medicaid is also the major payer for the care of the CMI in nursing homes. Unfortunately, however, the level of reimbursement is often very low. Not all states offer the total services allowed by the federal program, and care in free-standing psychiatric hospitals along with some specialized psychiatric nursing facilities is not permitted for the mentally ill, ages 22–64 years. Furthermore, only the very poor are eligible for Medicaid services. As a result, the program that reimburses the broadest array of community support and treatment services is available only to the poor.

The CMI, however, qualify in comparatively large numbers; an estimated 550,000 of the CMI are eligible for the Supplemental Security Income (SSI) program for the disabled poor, which entitles them to Medicaid in two-thirds of the states.[7] All of the states use a variety of criteria to qualify other individuals for Medicaid. On the average, the criteria of eligibility for Medicaid are income and assets at 50 percent of the federal poverty level. The CMI are disproportionately heavy users of the system of care. There are an estimated 35–45 million Americans who experience a mental disorder in the course of a year, accounting for approximately $20 billion in direct expenditures.[8] There are approximately 2.5 million Americans with chronic mental illness. Although those with chronic mental illness comprise only 5–7 percent of the mentally ill, they account for approximately $7.4 billion, or 37 percent of total direct costs. Those direct costs are divided among the specialty mental health sector ($4.236 billion), the general medical care sector ($2.498 billion), and the human services sector ($0.670 billion).[9]

The combined costs of direct services for the CMI are largely financed by government because the CMI are disabled and/or poor, which entitles them to government benefits. If approximately $3.7 billion in transfer costs—mostly associated with income support payments to the mentally disabled through SSI, SSDI, and the Veterans' Administration—are added to the direct care costs, the total is $11.1 billion. Approximately 59.5 percent of the total expenditures, including transfer payments, are from federal sources; 37.8 percent are from states; and only 2.7 percent are from local government.[10] In addition, approximately 70 percent of the resources under the control of state mental health authorities are devoted to the care of the CMI in institutional settings.

Problems In Organizing And Financing The System Of Care

The introduction of new payers and new programs into the system of services for the CMI has continued to divide public responsibility for their care. In an effort to return the care of the CMI to their local communities, the decentralization of services has further diffused public authority and accountability. From the turn of the century until the 1960s, the state government held centralized authority and responsibility for the CMI. Thereafter, responsibility has been a mix involving the federal government, state government, local government, and private providers. For example, care for a chronically mentally ill individual might be provided directly by the federal government through the Veterans' Administration or by local government through the county hospital. Or at that level the care might be financed by the federal Medicare program; by a federal block grant to a local community mental health center administered by the state; or by Medicaid, jointly funded by federal and state revenues. The complexity is exacerbated by the fact that about 125,000 individuals remain in beds in state mental hospitals on any given day.[11]

States are divided into regions, each served by a state hospital. However, these areas may not coincide with catchment area designations for federal community mental health centers. Cities and urban counties may be divided into more than a dozen such areas with no single city or county-wide authority responsible for the care of the CMI. Scarce, expensive, and/or innovative resources in one catchment area may not be available to the CMI residents of an adjacent community because of strict adherence to the catchment area concept. Similarly, duplicate services might go under-utilized in adjacent districts. Existing local government agencies are often inefficient and excessively bureaucratic, not only tied to rigid personnel and procurement mechanisms but also dependent on state and federal finances rather than locally-generated revenues.

Given such a complex and highly differentiated system of services, clinicians in a state-operated community mental health center, for example, might not know anything about additional care financed by Medicaid which was provided to a client in a private psychiatrist's office. Some patients receive duplicate prescriptions from the Veterans' Administration and the community mental health center then fail to follow up on care at either site. When such individuals present themselves in a crisis at the city hospital's emergency room, there is no knowledge of the patients' care history, and there will be no single individual or agency assigned primary responsibility for the client's treatment.

These situations are exacerbated by a system of financing which distributes limited resources unevenly under a perverse system of incentives. Financing mechanisms tend to favor institutional care over non-institutional services, as well as acute treatment services over long-term care and rehabilitation services. Hospital care, although critical to the system of services, is probably overused because more efficient alternatives are not financed. Disability benefits may continue for decades, while potential beneficiaries are denied access to vocational rehabilitation programs. Reimbursements tend to favor acute patients whose treatment is more circumscribed and of shorter duration than the complex medical/psychiatric/social welfare services needed by the CMI. This has become especially true in an era of payment and provider risk-sharing arrangements in which the CMI are perceived as "bad risks." Historically, the system of financing has discriminated against the CMI. Although this remains true, some innovative services, especially in the Medicaid program, have been designed specifically to meet the needs of the CMI.

Contemporary Solutions

Beginning in the 1970s, the National Institute of Mental Health (NIMH) sponsored the Community Support Program (CSP), which advocated services for the CMI through revitalized responsibility at the state and local levels.[12] CSP refocused attention on the CMI as the number one priority for public mental health resources, accepting the current needs of the CMI as preeminent over preventing chronicity through early treatment of acute problems. CSP developed the concept of a community support system as a "network of caring" bolstered by ten essential components which included housing and case management, as well as more traditional health and mental health services. CSP also promoted the idea of a core service agency, a single source of accountability in the service system to accept responsibility for CMI clients. The concepts caught on with many states. Each state modified the concepts and components to meet local needs and to fit local budgets. Ultimately, states poured considerably greater resources into community support programs than the initial NIMH investment of $6 million in grants.[13]

Although CSP was a start, it was not sufficient to meet the growing problem of the care of the CMI in America's largest cities. Many of the problems already discussed have remained unchanged in spite of CSP intervention in the 1970s and early 1980s. Nothing brought the continuing problem of the care of the CMI into sharper focus than the problem of the homeless.

Building on concern about the homeless mentally ill, the newest innovation in the organization of care for the CMI has been sponsored by The Robert Wood Johnson Foundation (RWJF) in conjunction with the United States Department of Housing and Urban Development. This program attempts to centralize responsibility for the urban CMI under mental health authorities which assume clinical, administrative, and fiscal responsibility for them.[14]

There are many models for providing centralized fiscal responsibility which have been learned from innovative state and local governments. Some mental health authorities are direct providers of mental health services. Other authorities are developing more sophisticated mechanisms for contracting with provider organizations, including specifications for obtaining measurable outcomes in performance contracts and for negotiating agreements competitively. Some authorities have developed specific incentive contracts which reward providers for using fewer hospital days than a selected historic target level in an effort to shift resources from institutions to community services.[15] Others are learning to use existing Medicaid benefits more flexibly to provide services in new types of settings, such as psychosocial rehabilitation clubs or community residences, and for new types of services, such as case management.

Any provision of services involves a contract between a payer and a provider. When the mental health authority provides services directly, it is under a contract with the public body that appropriates its budget. When the authority contracts out for a service, it purchases the service from the provider. Authorities and their clients may also seek payment from third parties, such as Medicaid, under a three-way contract among the parties.[16]

Provision of services by a mental health authority requires the largest initial investment in service capacity but insures control over services. Contracting out takes many forms, each suited to particular circumstances. For example, competitive bidding for contracts works best when there are multiple providers in a community. Some agreements, called performance contracts, require that units of performance be measured and monitored. Such conditions often cannot be met in the care of the CMI. Third-party financing in a free market approach to services works best when clients are informed consumers capable of shopping among providers. The indigent CMI often are not capable of taking advantage of the freedom of third-party benefits, and many of the benefits are so limited that the CMI are not attractive to providers. Each community must select the mix of financing mechanisms that is most efficient and protective of the interests of the CMI and that preserves the contract of trust among the authority, the public, the CMI, and their families.

The most innovative new financing mechanism proposes single-stream funding of services under the direct control of the local mental health authority. Modified versions of this approach have been in place in California, Wisconsin, Michigan, and Ohio. In this model, county government or a county mental health board receives an allotment of state and federal resources to combine with locally-generated resources (in Ohio as much as 25 percent of the total) to pay for all services for the CMI, including days of inpatient care at the state mental hospital. Some such local regions (within Rhode Island, Arizona, and New York) have attempted capitated approaches to mental health services for the CMI.[17] In these single-stream approaches, the local authority is at risk for all of the care for the CMI. It remains to be seen if this risk creates too strong an incentive for under-treatment rather than efficiency.

As with the centralized authorities themselves, many of these mechanisms are new and under evaluation and investigation. Soon, we may know if these well-intended innovations actually work. For now, the many service and financing demonstrations point in new directions that are generating interest across the United States. These directions may also be useful to other nations facing the dilemma of organizing and financing community-based care for individuals with chronic mental illnesses.

Notes

1. S. Grob, *Mental Illness and American Society*, 1875–1940 (Princeton: Princeton University Press, 1983).
2. H. Foley, S. Sharfstein, *Madness and Government: Who Cares for the Mentally Ill?* (Washington, D.C.: American Psychiatric Press, 1983).
3. E.M. Gruenberg, J. Archer, "Abandonment of Responsibility for the Seriously Mentally Ill," *Health and Society/Milbank Memorial Fund Quarterly* 57 (Fall 1979),485–506.
4. H. Goldman and R. Manderscheid, "Chronic Mental Illness in the United States," in R. Manderscheid and S. Barrett's *Mental Health—United States, 1987*, DHHS Publication No.(ADM) 87–1518 (Washington, D.C.: USGPO, 1987).
5. S. Sharfstein and H. Goldman, "Financing the Medical Management of Mental Disorders," *American Journal of Psychiatry*, 146 (1989), 345–49.
6. H. Goldman, C. Taube and S. Jencks, "The Organization of the Psychiatric Inpatient Services System," *Medical Care Supplement* 25 (1987), S6–S21.
7. Goldman and Manderscheid.
8. R.G. Frank and M.S. Kamlet, "Direct Costs and Expenditures for Mental Health Care in the United States in 1980," *Hospital and Community Psychiatry*, 36 (1985), 165–8.
9. H. Goldman and R. Frank, "Evaluating the Cost of Chronic Mental Illness," from Conference on the Economics of Disability (Washington, D.C., 1985).
10. B. Dickey and H. Goldman, "Public Health Care for the Chronically Mentally Ill: Financing Operating Costs. Issues and Options for Local Leadership." *Administration in Mental Health*, 14, No. 2 (1986), 63–77.

11. R. Manderscheid and S. Barrett, Mental Health—United States, 1987, DHHS Publication No. (ADM) 87–1518 (Washington D.C.: USGPO, 1987).

12. J. Turner and W. TenHoor, "The NIMH Community Support Program: Pilot Approach to a Needed Social Reform," *Schizophrenia Bulletin* 4, No. 3 (1978).

13. R.C. Tessler and H.H. Goldman, *The Chronically Mentally Ill—Assessing Community Support Systems* (Cambridge: Ballinger, 1982).

14. L.H. Aiken, S.A. Somers and M.F. Shore, "Private Foundations in Health Affairs: A Case Study of the Development of a National Initiative for the Chronically Mentally Ill," *American Psychologist* 41 (1986), 1290–5.

15. R.G. Frank and H.H. Goldman, "Financing Care of the Severely Mentally Ill: Incentives, Contracts, and Public Responsibility," *Journal of Social Issues* 45, No. 3 (1989), 131–44.

16. Ibid., 131–44.

17. C. Taube and H. Goldman, "State Strategies to Restructure Psychiatric Hospitals: A Selective Review," *Inquiry* 26 (1989), 146–56.

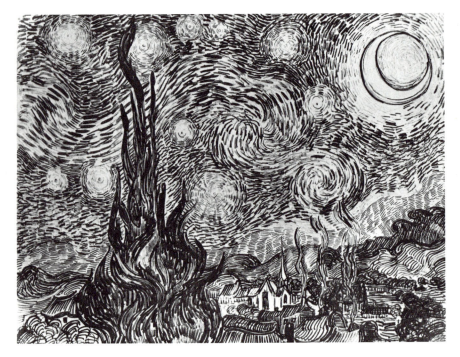

Cypresses Under the Night Sky. Painting, Vincent Van Gogh, 1890; Courtesy of The Bettmann Archive.

∽ INTO THE 1990s: THE FUTURE OF COMMUNITY MENTAL HEALTH SERVICES IN BRITAIN
An Introduction to Collected Conference Papers from England

By Helen Smith

These background papers provide a "snapshot" of current views and good practices in the major areas of British mental health services.

This overview begins with a brief outline of the history and major policy initiatives in the mental health field. This is followed by a detailed look at the government's latest white paper on community care which describes the continuation of the radical transformation of services for people with long-term needs. Hospital and community resettlement practices are then described, followed by three major aspects of mental health care—housing, crisis services, and work opportunities. People who use services need assistance in obtaining a package of care to meet their needs, so different models of case management are represented. Service users constantly seek a collective voice to make their needs known, and the section on self-advocacy traces this welcome development. People from minority groups have special needs for an ethnically sensitive service, and these issues are explored in more detail.

The environment of mental health services is changing rapidly. Because of this, training, research, and evaluation are essential to ensure that newly developed services are actually needed and wanted by the people who will be using them.

A section on services for people with challenging behavior has not been included. This is partly due to our current lack of expertise and imagination in finding ways of supporting this small group of people. There are too few examples of good practice, although we are now starting to learn from the great progress made through services for people with learning difficulties and challenging behavior. There is also a feeling that people with challenging behavior should expect the same things from a service as other people with long-term needs, the only difference being the level of staff support needed to live in ordinary housing, maintain employment, and make friends. In this sense, all that follows in this collection of papers applies equally to people with challenging behavior.

Given the brevity of these papers, they are, indeed, only "snapshots", but hopefully they will communicate the direction and the dynamism that characterizes services in England today.

✑ POLICY AND POLITICAL CONTEXT

By Simon Whitehead

Prior to 1800, most people with serious mental health problems—then known as lunatics—remained with their families, sometimes with financial support provided under the Poor Law. Those without families were confined to workhouses if they could not fend for themselves, while others who committed crimes ended up in prison. The only special facilities were private madhouses funded by wealthy families for their relatives and a very small number of hospitals funded through public donations.

The pressure for social reform that emerged as part of the industrial revolution led to the County Asylum Act of 1808. This required every county to provide an asylum, many of which are still in use today. Their numbers and size increased in the latter half of the nineteenth century as Poor Law guardians were encouraged to use them rather than workhouses. Hospitals originally built for one hundred people ended up housing 1,000 or more. Although admissions were restricted in the 1890 Lunacy Act, the existence of such a convenient and apparently respectable way of dealing with antisocial behavior fostered intolerance of deviant behavior in the community.

The early part of the nineteenth century saw the beginnings of a change in attitude. Certified confinement was increasingly challenged as the only solution to the problem of mental illness. The Maudsley Hospital in London began to demonstrate the possibilities of voluntary treatment in or out of the hospital. The 1930 Mental Treatment Act replaced the terms "asylum" and "lunatic" with "hospital" and "patient" and gave local authorities the power to set up services in the community. This led to a rapid increase in the use of out-patient clinics, and within eight years, 35 percent of hospital admissions had become voluntary. However, local authorities made very little use of their new powers, and services were still medically led and based on the large hospitals.

The creation of the National Health Service in 1946 did little in itself to improve matters. Local authority powers were extended, but people with mental illness or handicaps were given no priority. The National Health Service itself only spent 16 percent of its total budget on people with mental illness or handicaps and yet they occupied 42 percent of the beds. Major improvements did not occur until the 1950s, when the development of the phenothiazine group of drugs, which reduced the need for restraint, coincided with increasingly liberal attitudes. These arose from improvements in the overall standard of living and the advent of the welfare state.

The Development Of Community Care

Although services had sought alternatives to hospitalization during the first half of the twentieth century, care in the community did not emerge as a concept until the Royal Commission examined mental health services between 1954–1957. This led to the 1959 Mental Health Act which removed the legal distinction between mental hospitals and other hospitals, advanced the use of voluntary treatment wherever possible, and gave local authorities the responsibility to provide day and residential services in the community. In 1960, Enoch Powell, the Minister of Health, delivered a famous speech giving first indications that the days of the old asylums were numbered. This was in the context of a new hospital plan that sought to redefine the role of hospitals.

The idea that large institutions should be phased out and replaced by modern facilities in general hospitals and by community-based alternatives made little progress in the 1960s and early 1970s. While the number of people in psychiatric hospitals was reduced, little thought was given to what form a community psychiatric service should take or what services it should provide. As a result, the government published a white paper in 1975 entitled "Better Services for the Mentally Ill." It sought to identify the targets for the transition from the current hospital-dominated model towards a more community-oriented one. It was not backed by legislation, nor were new resources provided to accomplish the transition. However, it formally recognized the shift towards the concept of care in the community for people with mental health problems.

Joint Planning And Collaboration

Local authorities in the United Kingdom (County Councils, Metropolitan Boroughs, and District Councils) are responsible for providing social services, public housing, and public services in the community. Regional and district health authorities are responsible for all hospital services and, more recently, for all community-based health services. The role of local authorities has always been recognized as important in providing community mental health services; yet by the early 1970s, the extent of local community-based services was very limited.

In 1974, health service reorganization clearly separated the functions and responsibilities for health from local authority. In order to promote cooperation across the newly established boundaries, the government instituted joint planning and consultation mechanisms that required each area health authority and the local authorities in its territory to establish two joint bodies. The first was a Joint Consultative Committee (JCC) with members elected by the local authority and appointed by the health authority. The second was a Joint Care Planning Team (JCPT) where officers would meet. The JCPT was to be accountable to the JCC and the advisory JCC was accountable to the local government officials.

Perhaps because both health and local authorities were busy grappling with their new responsibilities and it was a period of increasing public expenditure as well, the joint planning process was not taken very seriously. In 1977, a financial incentive was created to encourage joint planning. Money was top-sliced from health allocations and made available as joint funds that could only be used on community alternatives to hospital care by agreement between health authorities. There was, however, great uncertainty and disagreement about how to spend this money. Mental health services were still accorded low priority by the local authorities, and few health authorities, which had continued to fund hospital services, had taken any positive initiatives in planning community services. Authorities did not perceive a need to plan jointly, and there was no community-based policy leadership. As public expenditure began to contract in the late seventies, there was little enthusiasm to pick up the costs of new services to be funded by a financial incentive that was only short-term.

Care In The 1980s

The 1975 government white paper had set out a model for the planned development of services. By the early 1980s, a number of other events increased the momentum for change. The 1980 Nodder Report on the organization and management problems of mental hospitals drew attention to the need for multi-disciplinary involvement in the assessment, treatment, and rehabilitation of individuals. At the same time, the concept of normalization had traveled across the Atlantic, and had begun to offer people involved in mental health services a value-based framework within which to consider service development. The growth of the civil rights and consumer movements in the United States also influenced thinking. For instance, a national voluntary organization called MIND became increasingly prominent in representing the interests of those suffering from mental illness as well as their families.

These factors combined to give greater priority to the closing of long-stay hospitals and increased pressure for the development of new acute hospital facilities with appropriate residential day treatment and personal support services in the community. By 1983, the Department of Health and Social Security issued a circular following a document for discussion entitled "Care in the Community." It extended the use of joint finance in order to encourage much greater collaboration between the statutory agencies. This circular also recognized the importance of voluntary agencies, education, and public housing services in the development of alternatives to long-stay hospital care. A new mental health act was passed in the same year that extended the restrictions on compulsory detention and treatment, broadened the concept of guardianship, and prescribed the clear need for joint assessment and rehabilitation processes for individuals.

Now that mental health services had become priority services, it was clear that government expected progress on the closing of the large hospitals. By 1985, disappointment in results prompted the Parliamentary Select Committee to publish a report. The committee, consisting of a multi-partisan group of members of parliament, reported that the move to care in the community was, at best, patchy. In particular, they found little forward progress in mental health services, very likely due to a lack of joint planning and service development. Worst of all, they identified a move to discharge patients from long-term care into inadequate, often unsupported alternatives in local communities. The reasons for this were many, but resulted from a lack of agreement within professions about what was needed; rivalry between professions; lack of commitment to joint planning from health and local authorities; and the lack of investment in alternatives to hospitals. These findings were confirmed a year later by the Audit Commission in a report on joint planning. They identified confusion and lack of progress drawing particular attention to the problems inherent in multi-agency involvement where no one agency has overall responsibility for guiding service development.

Current Issues

The 1985 and 1986 government reports confirmed the fears of a number of health professionals and relatives of people with severe mental illnesses that care in the community was failing. While many have been discharged from the hospitals and new services have developed in some areas, undoubtedly new developments have often neglected the needs of people with more serious mental health problems. Because of the people discharged from the hospital without adequate support and the large numbers still remaining in hospitals, care in the community is not perceived as an effective alternative. Even though there are instances of good practice that show what can be achieved, we need to understand why the field of mental handicap, such as retardation for example, has shown greater progress than that of mental illness.

Most people with mental health problems do live in their own homes in the community, but services have continued to be dominated by a single health agency operating like a large institution. Although the importance of community-based local services has been discussed since 1930, their development has been accorded very low priority and provision is poor in quantity and quality. With the heavy emphasis on the medical dimension of mental health, the social aspect has been neglected. This has been fueled by the stigma attached to mental illness and the continuing public fear of "madness" and "mad people" evoking little pity or understanding.

As mentioned, one of the principal factors in the very patchy development of community mental health care has been the lack of policy leadership. The Department of Health has always interpreted its policy role as a very generalized one, expressed in terms of trimming down the size of the large old hospitals and developing adequate alternatives. The department has not involved itself with defining what these alternatives should be, instead leaving that to health and local authorities and other agencies. This policy responsibility would work if there was agreement at a local level, but collaboration has always been poor. In the sixties and early seventies, community social workers were very influenced by the anti-psychiatry movement and tended to react against the medical domination of psychiatric services. Psychiatry, in turn, reacted to what it perceived as hostility to the profession. Although the numbers of patients in psychiatric hospitals dwindled in the 1970s, new long-term patients emerged and psychiatrists asserted dominance by holding onto the beds that symbolized their power. The nursing profession responded in both ways, with part of the nurses committed to the long-stay hospitals while others recognized the opportunities of a community-based service backed by the use of modern drugs.

There are many exceptions to this simplistic analysis, but the lack of any consensus about what form a community-based service should take, if any, has been central to the slow development of alternatives to hospitals. The importance of a value-based approach has been recognized in the field of mental handicap, where considerably more success has been achieved through value-based policy leadership bringing together disparate professional groups and agencies to form one view about the direction and nature of services required. This leadership has been aided by the introduction of general management of the health service which assigns responsibility to one person for ensuring that there is both a policy and a plan. The task of bringing together the opposing voices and attitudes in the mental health field, on the other hand, has proved daunting and much more complex than originally envisioned.

Finally people involved in the psychiatric services are speaking out and becoming involved. The beginnings of this change go back to the early seventies but did not gather momentum until more recently when recognition was given to the importance of individualizing services. As professionals and care managers started to adopt a value-based approach to support, including an individual's own wishes and needs, then the relevance of supportive user groups, patients' councils, and advocacy services grew. The movement has not progressed in the strong separatist way that has been the experience in some parts of the United States, but more through partnership and negotiation with professionals and managers of services. There is now hope that the wider involvement of service users in decisions affecting them will make service developments more relevant and more appropriate.

The political and policy issues that will affect future developments are contained in the current government's plans for major changes in the way the national health service and social services are provided and delivered. By providing services that offer consumers choices that are more responsive and relevant to the needs of individuals, the government is seeking to use some of the principles of the marketplace to change the way services are accessed, planned, delivered, and paid for. Attempting to avoid the label of privatization, new organizations and systems will be instituted that will clearly separate the functions of strategic planning/purchasing from direct service provision and access to services through primary health care or case managers. The statutory agencies will be less involved in the direct service provision of social care. Such changes may offer exciting new opportunities but there is concern that they will not be enough. Effective community services will depend on clearly stated and shared values; shared commitment among users, providers, and purchasers; and the assurance of qualitatively sound opportunities for people with mental health problems to live as nearly normal lives as possible. The current changes offer no guarantees but may give us the tools to finally do the job right.

APPENDIX – CARING FOR PEOPLE: COMMUNITY CARE IN THE NEXT DECADE AND BEYOND

A White Paper by the British Government

This section is a summary of the key points in the white paper.

The Key Changes
Note that common designations are abbreviated as follows:
HA — health authority
RHA— regional health authority
LA — local authority
NHS— National Health Service

Local authority responsibility	Social services authorities to be responsible for assessing the social care needs of populations and individuals, designing and organizing the necessary services.
Purchase/provider separation	Social services authorities to purchase from their own directly managed services, from independent sector, and from voluntary organizations. A mixed economy.
Funding – transfers from social security – choice – disincentive	Social services authorities to receive social security funds currently paid to support individuals in private/voluntary residential and nursing homes. (Transitional protection.) Options exist to offer choice between residential/domiciliary. Local authorities "own" residents excluded from all social security entitlements.
Community care plans	Prepared by health and local authorities, each to consult the other. Desirability of joint plans. Plans to be scrutinized by social services inspectors/RHAs for content and evidence of achievement.

Individual care plans	Social services authorities to assess individual needs (with advice from HAs if needed), create care packages, appoint key workers. Review regularly.
Case management	Case managers to arrange assessment, use funds to purchase care packages, ensure regular review, work at local level.
Mental health grants	Targeted specific grants to be issued via regional and district health authorities to local authorities to fund community care for people with severe mental health problems.

The Context — Why Change Must Occur

Inequalities	Audit Commission (1986) showed uneven development of community care across the country.
Uncoordinated development	Health and local authorities pursuing separate agendas, inevitable gaps and overlaps, poor use of resources.
Who's in charge?	Lack of single responsible agency for community care allows selective interpretation and confusion for recipients. Place of general practitioner?
Inflexibility	Services more determined by what's available rather than individual need. Assessment of individual rare, review and reassessment rarer.
Perverse incentive	Social security support goes to recipients of residential/nursing home care without assessment of need or option of domiciliary care instead.
	Placement means no direct HA or LA financial responsibility—a perverse incentive to choose residential care solutions.

Relocation of long-term care	Value-driven efforts to reduce long-term care in hospitals to ensure better quality of life failing because of lack of shared priorities (HA/LA) and poor joint planning.
Demographic change	Expansion of frail elderly population (by 50 percent in 1984–93 for those over 85) demands new and better forms of community care.
Failure to separate case management from resource management	Managers, particularly in social services departments, faced confused objectives of running services and assessing individual needs.
Failure to combine therapeutic and prosthetic efforts for community care clients	Community care is not just about supporting people but also about improving their ability to cope.

Community Care for the Individual

Assessment	A personal consideration of individual need, arranged by the local authority using health staff where necessary.
The care package	Strong recommendation for care at home where possible. Emphasis on support which is practical, locally appropriate, developed with the client, and ensures the needs of caregivers considered.
Clear point of contact	A single responsible agency, a case manager and/or a key worker.
Referral	Can be via health authority, local authority, or self. Emphasis on role of general practitioner in identifying and passing on need to LA.
Choice	Less pressure for the institutional solution. Consultation in care package design. Information on help more widely available.

Tasks for the National Health Service

Define roles

In consultation with individual local authorities, clarify, where necessary, the content of community health services/overlaps with other providers.

Provide community health services

Ensure the contribution of district nurses, health visitors' therapy services, chiropody, dentistry, clinical psychology, and specialist health teams (mental health, learning difficulties, elderly, and disabled); offer assessment procedures and community care packages.

Hospital services

New discharge arrangements; hospital support for community care such as respite.

General practitioners and their teams

Arrangements to ensure their role in identification of need and their contribution to assessment and care packages.

Community health needs

Ensure that community health needs are identified and incorporated into community care plans.

Evaluation and monitoring

Contribute to the evaluation procedures for community care and to registration and monitoring of long-term care provision.

Mental health grants

Negotiate expenditure of targeted mental health grants with local authorities.

NHS long-term care

Provide long-term residential care for some people with major specialist health requirements. Secure alternative residential care in non-hospital locations for others in consultation with local authorities.

Areas for Collaboration

Planning
– LA community care
– mental health

Both agencies' plans must be prepared in consultation. Joint plans are the desirable outcome. New planning arrangements task oriented, time limited; planning agreements emphasized. Plans to be monitored by SSI for LAs; by RHAs for HAs.

Opportunities for Better Community Care

Case management

With key workers, offers opportunities for community care patients/clients to know who is in charge; for best use of local resources; for less emphasis on residential solutions.

The move away from long-term in hospitals

Clarification of need for hospital long-term care, and for alternatives for those who do not need hospitalization. Requires shared objectives and collaboration HA/LA. Application of mental health grants.

The role of caregivers

A new set of principles to ensure consultation involvement and information for informal caregivers.

Workforce

More patient/client-related emphasis. Changing roles for professionals. New jobs as care managers/key workers. New skills needed in assessment, multidisciplinary cooperation, identifying community health needs.

If We Fail

To define roles of HA/LA in community care

Boundary disputes, inappropriate packages, wasteful use of trained staff.

To achieve joint plans based on agreed principles	Misuse of the free nature of health care to make LA community care cheaper.
	Failure to achieve acute-ward release because of lack of subsequent community support.
	Failure to relocate the care of people living inappropriately in long-stay hospitals.
To collaborate on the ground	Baffled consumers, alienated caregivers, unnecessary breakdown in domiciliary care, rising rate of institutionalization. Exhausted resources.

Major Concerns

The major concerns about the implementation of this otherwise welcome initiative are as follows:

(a) It is a massive change in funding, assessment of need and provision which will take time to be understood at local levels. It will take time to stimulate the range and variety of imaginative providers. Management must be optimistic and energetic but must be given time to experiment cautiously.

(b) Indicative strategies will be based on aggregates of assessed client needs. There will be more money to play with. The talk of it being a "poisoned chalice" with the delegation of blame to the local level for there not being enough resources is a dangerous attitude that may be used to excuse inefficiency and failure. There should be early public debate on the extent to which the local population should approve increases in the community charge to provide the standard of community care they believe right for their relatives, friends, and neighbors.

(c) The local authorities will need to recruit large numbers of very able individuals who will need training to be competent in handling budgets and allocating resources within defined localities in accordance with assessed needs. Also, the professional staff with responsibility for assessing a need will require careful selection and training. There are some really confused ideas about the local delivery system. It is even proposed, in one area, that those assessing need should hold budgets to purchase from a local arranger and contractor of services but the latter would have no line management control of the former. Local authorities have never delegated much to their senior managers and now there appears to be a risk that they will delegate too much, too quickly, too far down the hierarchy.

(d) The private sector and the voluntary sector need clear, well-thought out strategies if they are to respond imaginatively to the new challenges. There must be consistency and continuity in these plans. There will be a significant time lag before they can respond. Many local authority politicians seem to attach little importance to ensuring that the private sector has the incentive of reasonable levels of profit. The government needs to resolve the controversy over whether voluntary organizations contracting for services should be accountable to a statutory authority because many believe that such accountability compromises their advocacy role.

(e) The disincentive for local authorities to put pressure on health authorities to deliver social as well as health care because it is free will be a powerful deterrent to planning. This problem must be addressed openly in joint planning between local and health authorities. Because the funding of community care from both services starts from very different positions in different areas, there can be no general formula.

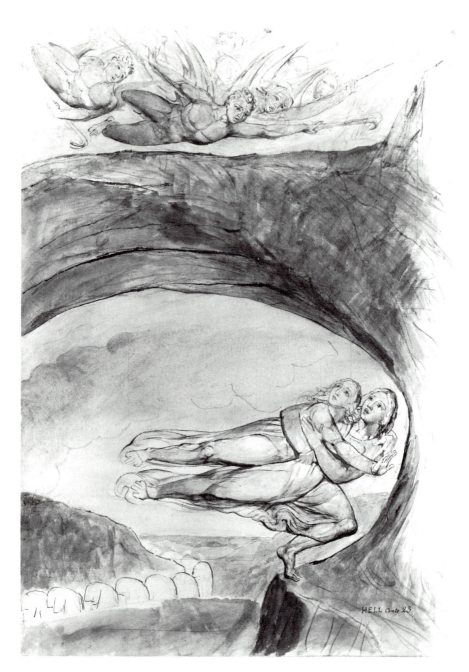

Virgil Rescues Dante from the Evil Demons. 18th–19th Century Watercolor, William Blake; Courtesy of the Fogg Art Museum, Harvard University, Cambridge, Mass.; Bequest of Grenville L. Winthrop.

THE COMMUNITY MENTAL HEALTH SERVICES AND WORK

By *Ann Davis*

Services promoting ordinary and valued lifestyles for people with long-term mental health problems must consider the issue of work. Studies consistently show that most mental health service recipients living in the community are unemployed.[1] In the United Kingdom, employment conveys important social and economic status. Being excluded from work and income has profound consequences. Work provides identity and self esteem. It gives structure to each day, as well as the opportunity for social life and friendship. It provides leisure with a greater meaning and can sometimes be a source of income.[2]

Many studies of health and unemployment in Britain in the 1970s and 1980s revealed the stress and mental health problems associated with periods of unemployment and the effects these have on individuals and their households.[3] A vicious cycle can arise. Loss of work triggers difficulties, and a history of mental illness along with use of mental health services raises substantial barriers to returning to employment.[4] Therefore, providing access to and opportunities for work are important mental health service components. It is important for service providers to identify the differentials of age, class, gender, ethnic experience, and work expectations, both paid and unpaid. Service providers must also acknowledge that work remains universally a key element for any individual, influencing one's feelings of self-worth and ability to cope with daily life.

These work-related challenges facing the recipients of mental health services are considerable and are unlikely to lessen in the 1990s. They arise not just from changes in mental health policy and service provision but from the introduction of two additional factors: high levels of unemployment in the United Kingdom and major changes in social security provision.

Work Programs And Unemployment

Until the early 1970s, the mental health service model was one of employment rehabilitation and resettlement through industrial therapy. It drew heavily on practices developed in the field of physical disability. This approach measured individual functioning in certain kinds of employment and provided time-limited training programs designed to improve that functioning. Some of these programs were in settings created by the state-funded disability employment services. People with mental health problems were always a minority group within this service. Such programs provided both open employment and sheltered employment opportunities. Other programs had a mental health base in hospital industrial therapy schemes or newly emerging day hospitals and centers. These programs were also designed to equip the individual with confidence and skills either to operate in a sheltered work environment or to enter open employment. At best the programs achieved these goals. At worst, they provided only boring, repetitive work in situations where contract completion dates dominated staff concerns at the cost of providing truly useful employment. The main recipients of these services were men admitted to hospitals. For the many women entering and leaving psychiatric hospitals, help was typically focused on the resumption of their roles as unpaid domestic workers and caregivers in their own households.

This powerful and progressive model broke the century-long tradition of using psychiatric patients in laundries, gardens, canteens, and hospital wards to maintain these inadequately staffed institutions to which they had been consigned for most of their adult lives. However, the success of the work rehabilitation and resettlement approach depended crucially on the availability of employment in wider society. The rapid increase in unemployment in the United Kingdom from the mid-1970s to the mid-1980s, coupled with over 1.5 million of the registered workforce being unemployed today, has undermined this model of good practice. While there were wide regional differences in unemployment rates, the change in employment climate was felt nationally. This affected groups with disabilities whose employability was critically dependent on the demand for labor. As unemployment rates soared, there was a marked increase in professional uncertainty and a loss of confidence in what could be achieved by traditional industrial therapy programs inside and outside the mental health field.

Social Security Changes

While the industrial therapy approach was being undermined by changes in employment opportunities, changes in social security provisions made it more difficult for mental health services to develop directions for work initiatives. In the 1970s, the government introduced several new benefits for people with disabilities and their caregivers. These increased the income available to people who could establish their incapacity for work. However, people with long-term mental health problems then found themselves in a position of financial loss if they actually developed their capacity for work.

The most recent major reforms in the state social security system in the United Kingdom have exacerbated this situation. The government's current concern is to wean people from dependency on state benefits and encourage them to take more responsibility for their own financial security. In pursuing this concern, government has sought to control the numbers on the unemployment register by making the social security criteria for work availability and incapacity tighter. The rationale is to target resources for the disabled while encouraging those capable of work to drop benefits and take employment on government work projects if private sector jobs are not available. The reality for people with long-term mental health problems is that maximum income benefits come through a declaration of sickness and disability. Considerable financial penalties are imposed on those who decide they wish to declare themselves as capable of and available for work. Such declarations result in cuts to weekly benefits based on means, as well as a return to low-paid employment typically available to marginal employment groups.

Losing social security benefits does not just result in less weekly income. Some of the innovative developments in mental health housing depend critically on recipients' claiming maximum social security payments. The loss or reduction of these payments by re-entry to work or a declaration of availability for work can, therefore, result in the loss of valued and supported accommodations because costs can no longer be met by the recipient.

Our current social security provision is at odds with the goals of mental health services striving to deliver flexible and individualized rehabilitation, resettlement, and integration to recipients. Yet this aspect of the perverse incentives of the social security system on community care policies has not been addressed in the recent white paper. Complex financial disincentives remain for the many individuals with mental health problems who wish to undertake training or work, both paid and voluntary.[5]

Work Initiatives In A Difficult Climate

These changes in social security provisions and mental health employment policies have left a very difficult climate in which to address the issues of both work and unemployment for people with mental health problems. Yet a number of initiatives have emerged in response to the strongly expressed wish of most mental health service recipients to remain working and productive members of society. Several are models of the best practice possible within existing constraints and point the way forward for the 1990s. A number of these schemes have generated a collective political lobby to change those employment and social security regulations considered to be undermining the development of better practice in the 1990s.[6]

It is difficult to single out similarities and differences between the small, scattered work initiatives striving for good practice. These schemes are commonly characterized by the determined efforts of committed professionals and recipients working creatively and opportunistically to deliver work opportunities and to maximize resources in spite of the constraints of local and national circumstances. These are precisely the "strong and committed local champions of change" that the Audit Commission Report noted as being "the single most important factor common to all successful community care initiatives."[7] Without imposing unwarranted coherence on this aspect of services, five broad approaches to providing work experience and enhancing access to employment can be identified as follows:

- Industrial therapy schemes within and outside mental health projects;
- Work schemes in open employment;
- Work opportunities in mental health projects;
- Voluntary work within and outside mental health projects; and
- Educational opportunities within and outside mental health projects.

Industrial Therapy In The 1990s

Despite current problems, many industrial therapy schemes have adapted to the changed economic climate by creating work opportunities that are an end in themselves. One example is a sheltered work experience that is not necessarily time-limited but provides recipients with the chance to reestablish work routines, increase social contact, and earn a little extra money each week within the limits of the social security benefit rules. These schemes can still fall into the trap of creating routine, passive, boring work substitutes. Schemes outside of the mental health services are primarily geared to the needs of people with physical disabilities. However, there have been one or two notable attempts to use this traditional work situation more actively and creatively for people with long-term mental health problems.

The Skills and Practical Activities Network (SPAN) based at Mapperley Hospital in Nottingham provides a service for approximately 150 people with long-term mental health problems—90 percent of whom live in the community. It has altered a traditional industrial therapy setting to create a therapeutic environment that taps peoples' strengths through a range of practical activities. It seeks to empower recipients who are members of the scheme to participate fully in all the decisions made in the project. Work which is intrinsically useful and income-generating is one component of the program. The overall program includes furniture repair and renovation, gardening, and printing. Its recycling project collects and renovates old bicycles. Alongside this activity are a variety of social, educational, and leisure opportunities which members organize. SPAN's approach emphasizes peoples' active achievements and, at the same time, offers help with the problems generated by such individual achievement. Therefore it combines traditional elements of a mental health service with active, income-generating activity by those who receive the service. Mapperley Hospital is scheduled to close in 1992. The plan is to bring SPAN to four local sites so that its ties with local communities are closer.

Work Schemes In Open Employment

The range of employment training schemes created by the government over the last decade is now the major source of alternatives to paid open employment for those registered as unemployed and available for work in the United Kingdom. These schemes are time-limited, targeted at both young people and the registered long-term unemployed, and they provide an income for those just above the social security benefit level. To date, the government has not taken any positive stance on the needs of people with mental health problems who are available for work. However, people with such problems are joining these programs to gain work experience and acquire skills. The most recent response of the Youth Training Scheme (compulsory for unemployed 16- and 17-years-olds) to the problems posed by young people with mental health problems has been to exclude them rather than to integrate them. Staff have been asked to guide young people displaying behavioral difficulties to obtain medical evidence of mental illness so that they can claim a disability-related benefit instead of seeking work experience and skill training.[8] A recent review of the main employment training scheme for adults claims that the high incidence of health problems among people who have been unemployed for over two years has actually been exacerbated by policies of community care for mental patients.[9]

Despite this lack of response through government employment schemes, some community-based mental health support services do help recipients who want to join employment schemes. Through individual support from preparation to travel and work routines, or detailed information about changing from benefit income to employment training allowances, these schemes enable a few individuals to make an informed choice. Such a plan may offer employment for up to a year, and may provide skills and experience that will enhance access to employment in the future.

Apart from government employment schemes, employers are offering individually negotiated plans to people with mental health problems. For example, a Christian-based workers cooperative in whole foods in Southampton offers such a work opportunity. The availability of this kind of arrangement depends on both the interest of local employers and the priority that mental health services give to identifying and canvassing for such opportunities. Experience suggests that there must be considerable enthusiasm and commitment from all parties concerned because of the employment and benefit hurdles that have to be overcome to ensure a secure and unstressed work opportunity for the recipient.

Work Opportunities in Mental Health Schemes

As mentioned, mental health day services do provide information and support for individuals moving toward work in open employment. At the same time, some services have also developed in-house work opportunities on a smaller scale than those in modified industrial therapy units. These developments have been a response to recipient demand as well as to the lack of local employment opportunities. To fund these enterprises, various schemes have combined existing health or social-service funding with supplements from charitable foundations, government employment services, and the local business communities. They have also tried to interpret benefit rules to provide the maximum income for recipients.

The Peter Bradford Trust is a voluntary organization that provides opportunities for about 85 people who have suffered a variety of disadvantages including mental health problems and years of institutional living. Alongside its housing provision, it has developed work opportunities for its recipients who claim social security benefits. The trust stresses worker involvement and satisfaction in providing work that is both well-organized and rewarding. It also seeks to create useful jobs, valued both by the workers and the wider community, and situations maximizing the contact between workers and the community. The main work scheme of the trust is furniture repair and restoration. This emphasis often links the trust with other related work opportunities.

Another voluntary work scheme is Many Hands, run by the Kensington and Chelsea Mental Health Association, which is housed among other small businesses in a commercial workshop. It provides training in marketable skills for people with long-term mental health problems. The project meets high expectations with standards required in open employment. Training courses include painting and decorating, carpentry, and office skills. Approximately eight trainees are accepted for each course. Individuals apply independently for advertised courses. Referrals or references from these mental health professionals are given consideration only after an informal interview. Course tutors are employed for their professional knowledge, and each trainee works at his or her own pace. Placements are made towards the end of each course, and some individuals move straight into open employment. Others join the project's own decorating and carpentry business agency which provides self-employment opportunities in the local community. Still others move into voluntary work. The leaders expect trainees to participate in weekly management meetings. Approximately 35 people use the project in any one year.

Voluntary Work Inside And Outside Of Mental Health Projects

Several mental health community projects encourage recipients to consider voluntary work as an alternative to paid employment. This often takes the form of befriending, visiting, or caring for others; or it draws upon skills such as typing, joinery, and plumbing to help organizations and individuals who cannot afford to pay for the service. Some schemes pioneer contacts with organizations offering opportunities for voluntary workers. Others encourage recipients to contact the local volunteers bureau for interviews and suitable work offers. Although this work is unpaid, there are still some issues of social security benefits to be resolved. For example, evidence of capacity to work can jeopardize ongoing payments of higher-rate disability benefits.

Services such as the North Derbyshire Mental Health Service Project create their own work opportunities through self-managing social groups that run the service and offer support to individuals. Those in this project take on a range of tasks such as a voluntary or paid worker might assume in a more traditional mental health service.

Educational Opportunities Inside And Outside Mental Health Projects

Some day services have increasingly helped recipients to acquire interests and skills through local adult education and training. The usual approach is to encourage individuals to enroll in available courses and then to offer help as they go through the programs. Some services build an interim step by arranging for a group to go through an educational course together with a tutor or by making classroom arrangements for the group with a local college. Decisions need to consider recipients' needs and levels of confidence as well as the availability of local resources. The varied courses include such subjects as basic literacy, creative writing, further qualifications, and practical skills such as car maintenance, photography, and woodworking.

As part of its approach and philosophy, the North Derbyshire Mental Health Project provides self-managing recipient groups with independently controlled budgets to purchase selected training or leisure educational opportunities. This has changed the range of both individual and group ventures and achievements in the educational field. Some of these ventures have led individuals into employment or fields of further education and training.

Expanding Work Opportunities In The 1990s

In expanding employment in the 1990s, many creative, small-scale ventures constructively addressed an issue at the top of most service recipients' agendas. However, it continues to occupy a low priority on the service agendas of most professionals. The lessons learned during the last decade or so suggest that initiatives of this kind must be developed around interests of the individuals using the service as well as the characteristics of the local economy and its resources. This suggests that projects developing their own in-house experiences should think small and flexibly and be responsive to outside contacts and demands. They should harness business and employment knowledge to an enterprise focused on the mental health aspects of work and employment. The active involvement and participation of recipients in the organization and management of the project is crucial. Services developing work opportunities in the 1990s also need to keep up-to-date employment information on a changing situation both nationally and locally.

Good ideas and directions for the 1990s can be found within our existing services. However, to capitalize on them more systematically, there must be some changes in the wider employment service and social security provision. Such changes must promote work activity and employment as part of mental health rehabilitation rather than to constrain and undermine it. A recent government paper suggests that further changes in benefits for people with disabilities will be introduced in the early 1990s.[10] These include a benefit linked to employment. In its current form, this proposal is no more than a partial response to the issues of work and income facing people with mental health problems. It will have to be developed more comprehensively, and it must consider the costs of other services in this field if it is going to secure a better climate for the growth of work initiatives as an essential element of community mental health services.

Notes

1. N. Goldie, "I Hated it There, but I Miss the People," Health and Social Services Unit Research Paper 1, South Bank Polytechnic (London, 1988) and C. Legg and A. Kay, "Discharge to the Community: A Review of Housing and Support in London for People Leaving Psychiatric Care," *Good Practices in Mental Health* (1986).
2. R. Grover, "Workschemes at the Peter Bedford Trust," (1987) and Croom Helm, "Living after Mental Illness: Innovations in Services."
3. J. Popay, Y. Dhooge, and C. Shipman, "Unemployment & Health: What Role for Health & Social Services?" (London: Health Education Council, 1986).
4. A. Birch, "What Chance Have We Got? Occupation and Employment After Mental Illness—Patients' Views," (Manchester: MIND, 1983).
5. A. Davis and J. Betteridge, "Cracking Up: Mental Health Users' Experiences of Social Security," (MIND, 1990).
6. Employment Rehabilitation Consortium, details available from "Good Practices in Mental Health" (London).
7. Audit Commission. "Making a Reality of Community Care," (London: HMSO, 1986).
8. "Benefits for Young People with Behavioral Problems," a training agency draft letter to principal careers officers, (July, 1989).
9. Working Brief, November 1989 Unemployment Unit (London).
10. "The Way Ahead: Benefits for Disabled People," (London: HMSO).

Projects Mentioned In The Text

S.P.A.N., Mapperley Hospital, Porchester Road, Nottingham NG3 6AA

PETER BEDFORD TRUST, Legard Road, Highbury, London N5 1DE

MANY HANDS Unit, 2 & 3, Acklam Workshops, 10 Acklam Road, London W10 5QZ

NORTH DERBYSHIRE MENTAL HEALTH PROJECT, Chesterfield Community Center, Tontine Road, Chesterfield, Derbyshire

ASSESSING THE QUALITY OF COMMUNITY MENTAL HEALTH SERVICES

By Roger Blunden

In Britain, increasing emphasis is being given to assessing the quality of community mental health services. A recent government white paper on community care states:

> Securing and safeguarding the necessary quality of services must be a central objective for all agencies involved in the delivery of community care. People in need of community care are vulnerable and their interests should be protected.

> Clarifying responsibilities, establishing where accountability for service delivery lies, and specifying service requirements for contracts, will all help to keep attention focused on the quality and suitability of services. The government proposes to take a number of steps to be able to satisfy itself that authorities have plans in line with national objectives, and to monitor performance against those plans.[1]

While the importance of service quality is now recognized, there is little evidence thus far that attaining and monitoring quality is a prominent feature in existing services. There are, perhaps, two main reasons for this: first, very little consideration has been given so far to the definition of service quality; and second, organizations commissioning and providing services have generally not thought out the mechanisms for monitoring quality as a routine service feature.

This paper contains a brief discussion of these issues, together with some indication of the direction of quality assessment and implementation in Britain.

Defining Service Quality

Service quality can be defined both in terms of process and outcome. Process measures typically examine the usage and flow of services such as bed occupancy, admission and discharge rates, and length of stay. Less frequently, quality is assessed in terms of consumer satisfaction with the services received.[2]

Outcome measures include psychiatric diagnosis and changes in diagnosed morbidity. There is increasing movement toward evaluating services in terms of the quality of life of service users. Analysis of quality of life, particularly for dependent populations, is provided by John O'Brien[3] who identifies five components of a socially valued life as follows:

First, **community presence** is an individual's location within a community setting. Access to other people in a range of community settings, such as shops, leisure facilities, and places of education and employment, is a prerequisite for a satisfactory quality of life.

Relationships are a second crucial aspect of quality of life. Most people rely heavily on a range of relationships with friends, family members, colleagues, and peers.

Choice, a third important component of quality of life, includes small, everyday decisions such as what to eat or what to wear, and extends to major life decisions such as where to live or work and with whom. A major part of social existence involves the exercise of rights—for example, a citizen's right to vote and the right to refuse to engage in particular activities.

Fourth, **competence** requires basic abilities in communication, mobility, self-help, and social and leisure skills in order to participate fully in everyday activities.

Fifth, **respect** is, perhaps, dependent on the attainment of each of the other components. It is difficult to imagine a high quality of existence that does not involve a role worthy of the respect of others.

These five issues are particularly important in the context of community services. Are service users encouraged to have a wide circle of friends and acquaintances outside of service structures? Are they helped to form relationships with non-disabled people? Is there an active program to enhance competence in basic skills that will enable them to participate more fully in community life? Does the service present its users to the local community as valued citizens deserving respect? In Britain, some attempt is now being made to assess service quality in terms of broad quality of life variables, such as those outlined above. For example, some mental health services are now using the PASS[4] system to review their impact on users' quality of life.

Measuring And Achieving Service Quality

While there is growing acceptance of quality of life as a key outcome of mental health services, progress has been slow in developing adequate quality control systems. Interestingly, the quality issue is prominent among commercial organizations and the business community. Recently, many writers have addressed the problem of how manufacturing and service organizations can effectively meet their customers' needs.[5] The advice given and lessons drawn from these accounts of successful businesses appear relevant to developing effective services for people with mental health problems.

One major lesson is that successful organizations demonstrate a clear value system and devote considerable energy to actively promoting those key values at all levels. The values emphasize outcome rather than process. The successful organization has a well-defined notion of what it is trying to achieve. These achievements form the focus of attention. Organizations promoting core values as measured by client outcomes are then in a position to hold their staffs accountable, and they can build in mechanisms to review quality and take appropriate action.

Two further important features emerge from the literature on quality within organizations. One is sensitivity to the needs of the consumer. Organizations with a reputation for quality maintain close links with their customers. Everyone from senior management down, spends discussion time with customers, ensuring that the organization is receptive and responsive to customer views. Thus, the current move in Britain to closely involve mental health patients in service planning and monitoring may be one important step toward achieving quality.

Another feature of successful organizations is commitment to action and innovation. With commitment, there is an expectation that new ideas will be tested in practice and that some of these may fail. This allows the organization to be alive and developing rather than stagnating. Where unfulfilled consumer needs are identified, action is taken to meet the needs. This action orientation is an important part of the quality circle approach in industry in which small groups of workers are encouraged to identify problems, formulate solutions, and put these into practice.[6]

The work of the Independent Development Council is a recent attempt in Britain to make these ideas on quality operational in the field of human services.[7] According to this approach, a quality action group, comprising service users, staff, and other key stakeholders, is formed with a specific mission to examine service quality and to take appropriate action. The group first clarifies the values within which the service operates and the important outcomes in terms of clients' quality of life. A review and action process is begun. The group then focuses on one or more ways in which the service intends to benefit clients' lives. It collects evidence to evaluate how successful the service is in this area. After review, specific goals are set to improve the effectiveness of the service. The process is then repeated by identifying other client outcomes and initiating further reviews and action. The University of Bristol is currently investigating the applicability of this particular process to a range of services, including those for people with mental health problems.

Service Evaluation

Evaluation research is beginning to address some of the issues outlined above. Service evaluators are becoming concerned with methods of measuring client outcomes, and with ways of ensuring that the evaluation process is relevant to the development of better services. A recent research development is worthy of mention. This approach[8] helps evaluators decide whether conducting an evaluation is worthwhile. It asks whether key issues have been thought through sufficiently to ensure that the results of an evaluation could be used effectively.

There are seven important questions about evaluation to be asked in the early stages of planning such a service which are as follows:

- How is the service defined?

Most services in the health or social field are a complex mixture of components. For example, there may be various forms of therapy, treatment or counseling as well as managerial and administrative components. There may also be screening and case-finding procedures. Is the evaluation to be concerned with all of these by answering a question such as "How effective is our service as a whole?" Or are particular components of greater interest such as "How effective is our use of Bloggs's therapy techniques?"

There may also be uncertainty about what is and what is not a part of the service under review. For example, in evaluating a community residential service, what other components of the local service system are also included—social work support, day services, transport arrangements, social security benefits, or acute treatment?

- What does the service achieve for its users?

Service goals are often surprisingly difficult to state clearly. Sometimes there is no statement of aims at all. In other situations, aims are stated in terms of the services to be provided rather than their effect on users, such as whether to provide a day service, to provide support, to manage challenging behavior, or to provide training. Sometimes service aims are so vague that they are almost useless as a basis for an evaluation.

If a service is to be evaluated in terms of its effectiveness, it is essential to have a clear statement of the ways that users can benefit; for instance, living in an ordinary house in the community and participating in a range of community activities; learning and using new independence skills; obtaining and holding down a job; or making more use of local leisure facilities. Such statements arguably will help shape the design of the service and, perhaps, give staff a clearer sense of what they are setting out to achieve.

- Can client outcomes be measured?

If the service is to be evaluated in terms of its impact, it will be essential to have some measurement of client outcome. This might include information from service records, assessment forms, surveys, direct observations, test results, checklists, or a range of other measurement instruments. Again, a clear way of assessing effectiveness may be invaluable to those planning and designing the service.

- Does the service design logically lead to these client outcomes?

There are two potential problems with service design. First, the design may be totally inappropriate for achieving its stated aims. For example, a hospital or hostel-based residential service may be incapable of enabling its users to live independently in the community if the necessary community resources have not been included in the service design. In this case, there is a mismatch between the stated aims and the design format.

The second problem is less obvious and perhaps more common in human services. It occurs when the stated aims of the service are really beyond its scope. The service may only provide a small portion of the help its users actually need. For example, a rehabilitation service may aim to enable hospital residents to live independently in the community. However, it may only provide a limited amount of skill training in the hospital and may have little or no control over finding suitable accommodations and providing community support. A day service may include finding jobs for service users within its aims, but may not be geared to negotiating with employers or providing support in the workplace.

- What decisions will result from the evaluation?

It is often agreed that service evaluation is a good thing, but there may be considerable uncertainty about who is the customer for the evaluation and what that person or organization will do with the results once it is completed. Unless there is a clear reason for conducting the evaluation, the chances are that the results will lead to an interesting discussion but then be confined to the filing cabinet and quietly forgotten.

Still, there is considerable potential for the role of evaluative research in improving services. Results that might emanate from an evaluation include: deciding whether or not to continue funding a service; deciding on the level of resources to be made available; reviewing the overall direction of the service; or changing specific aspects of the service in order to make it more effective.

- Who can ensure useful results from the evaluation?

If the evaluation is treated as an afterthought, people whose participation is essential to the exercise are either not involved or are approached at too late a stage in the process. This may include service managers and staff, service users, or users' families who will play key roles in enabling evaluation to take place. Managers and staff who unexpectedly find themselves the subject of an evaluation have, at their disposal, a number of ways to limit its scope and effectiveness. The cooperation of service users and their families may be crucial, and there may be real advantages to involving them in discussions at an early stage.

Planners and decisionmakers will also need to be involved at an early stage to ensure that they obtain sensible answers to the questions listed here. If outside researchers are to be involved, it is crucial to bring them in as soon as possible. Many powerful evaluation methods compare what happened before a new service was introduced with what happened afterwards. This power will be lost if no one thinks about the evaluation until after the service has been introduced.

One useful approach is to set up an evaluation task force representing all those people with a stake in the evaluation process. This form of collaborative evaluation has been particularly valuable when the exercise is conducted as a means of identifying ways of improving services.[9]

In conclusion, this paper has outlined some of the current issues in assessment and achievement of service quality. It has selectively included issues that may be useful to discuss between American and British workers. In both countries, issues of service quality are likely to become more important as mental health services come under increasing scrutiny and as more effective solutions are sought to problems which could once be hidden within institutions. In Britain, the advent of a more competitive service environment and the emerging notions of tendering and contracting for services present the opportunity to enhance service quality in our newly developing community mental health services.

Notes

1. "HMSO Caring for People: Community Care in the Next Decade and Beyond," Cm 849 (London: HMSO, 1989).
2. See, for example, J.K. Wing, "Principles of Evaluation," from J.K. Wing and A.M. Bailey, eds., *Evaluating a Community Psychiatric Service* (London: Oxford University Press, 1972).
3. J. O'Brien, "A guide to lifestyle planning," in B. Wilcox and G.T. Bellamy, eds., *A Comprehensive Guide to the Activities Catalog: An Alternative Curriculum for Youth and Adults with Severe Disabilities* (Baltimore, Maryland: Paul H. Brookes, 1987).
4. W. Wolfensberger and L. Glenn, *PASS 3: A Method for the Quantative Evaluation of Human Services* (Toronto: National Institute on Medical Retardation, 1975).
5. See, for example, T.F. Gilbert, *Human Competence: Engineering Worthy Performance* (New York: McGraw-Hill, 1978) and T.J. Peters and R.H. Waterman, *In Search of Excellence: Lessons from America's Best-Run Companies* (New York: Harper and Row, 1982).
6. D.L. Dewar, *The Quality Circle Guide to Participation Management* (Englewood Cliffs, New Jersey: Prentice-Hall, 1982).
7. Independent Development Council for People with Mental Handicap, "Pursuing Quality: How Good Are Services for People with Mental Handicap?" (1986) Available from IDC, 126 Albert Street, London NW1 7NF.
8. J.S. Wholey, "Evaluability Assessment," in L. Rutman, ed. *Evaluation Research Methods: a Basic Guide* (Beverly Hills: Sage Publications, 1977).
9. M.Q. Patton, *Practical Evaluation* (London: Sage Publications, 1982).

Pertinent Projects Within the United Kingdom

Camden Consortium
c/o Camden Association for
    Mental Health
Hacker Centre
Anglers Lane
LONDON NW5 3DG

Daily Living Programme
115 Denmark Hill
LONDON SE5 8AZ

London Alliance for
Mental Health
c/o Camden Association for
    Mental Health
Hacker Centre
Anglers Lane
LONDON NW5 3DG

London Borough of Camden
Social Services Department
c/o The Town Hall
Euston Road
LONDON NW1

MIND in Waltham Forest
Forest Community Project
Marshall Community Centre
388-392 High Road
Leyton
LONDON E10 6QE

Nottingham Patients Council
    Support Group
Nottingham Advisory Group
c/o MIND
NOTTINGHAM NG1 3HL

Peter Bedford Trust
Legard Road
Highbury
LONDON N5 1DE

Lynfield Mount Hospital
Heights Lane
Bradford
WEST YORKSHIRE BD9 6DP

Nafsiyat Limited
Therapy Centre
278 Seven Sisters Road
LONDON N4

Harrambee Housing Association
Soho House
362-364 Soho Road
Handsworth
BIRMINGHAM B21 9QL

Afro-Caribbean Mental Health
    Association
35-37 Electric Avenue
Brixton
LONDON SW9

Gateshead Case Management
    Service
Department of Social Services
Wycombe District Offices
Council Offices
Front Street
Wycombe
NEWCASTLE NE16 4EG

CHOICE
152 Camden Road
LONDON NW1

Fanon Project
Brixton Circle Project
33 Effra Road
LONDON SW2

North Derbyshire Mental Health
  Services Project
Chesterfield Community Centre
Tartine Road
Chesterfield
DERBYSHIRE

Main Street Mental Health
  Resource Centre
86 Main Street
SPARKBROOK B11 1RS

Survivors Speak Out
c/o 33 Lichfield Road
LONDON N5 1DE

CRISIS SERVICES

By *Christina Murphy*

Until recently, interest in services for people with long-term needs focused on different models of housing, purposeful occupation, and provision of support. Providing a service response in a crisis was less of an issue. With the move towards community care gathering momentum, crisis service is starting to take on a greater priority. Research and information on the needs of people with long-term mental health problems, such as the need to maintain contact with the community or the effects of hospitalization, significantly influence the type of crisis service that should be established. This paper describes three different models of crisis service in practice: a planned crisis house, a community mental health center with specific services for people with long-term needs, and a daily living support program.

A Theoretical Framework For People With Long-Term Needs

Theories of crisis intervention have often been applied to people who do not have serious mental health problems. G. Caplan, one of the most influential theorists, defines a crisis as an emotional upset encountered when a problem arises that cannot be resolved by usual means. Three phases can be identified. First, there is a rise in tension as the person recognizes the problem is not being solved; second, tension and anxiety become intolerable as internal resources are exhausted and outside help is sought; third, the crisis is resolved either positively through new ways of coping with the problem or negatively through reliance on "solutions" that will actually cause future problems such as alcoholism, for example. The second phase is the ideal time for intervention and help should be provided as soon as it is requested.[1]

There have been few attempts to develop a theoretical perspective for people with long-term needs, but one exception has been Farewell[2] who attempted to link theories of crisis intevention to practice for people with serious mental health problems by developing a theory that views subsequent crises as being related to the initial crisis suffered by the person. As far as people with long-term mental health problems are concerned, services have been influenced by theories about the damaging effects of institutionalization and the possible benefits of community- based service. An increasing awareness during the 1960s of the importance of social factors in precipitating hospitalization was also significant in developing ideas about crisis services.

From Theoretical Issues To Practical Issues

In practice, the term crisis intervention has been used to describe a variety of service models, most of which support the view that crisis is a turning point and that an appropriate intervention can either ameliorate potential negative results or lead to a positive outcome. Models of service described as crisis intervention have ranged from emergency psychiatric clinics or community mental health centers to those services developed rigorously in accordance with Caplan's theories.

A number of groups can be identified as providing crisis services. Ratna,[3] who was involved with one of the first intervention services, identified four types: those which do specialized work on a specific problem (rape crisis centers, Samaritans); walk-in centers providing assessment counseling and treatment (emergency assessment clinics); crisis services provided as part of a comprehensive psychiatric service (crisis intervention services catering to people with a variety of mental health problems); and professionals dealing with psychiatric crises (general practitioners and social workers). In addition, Newton has identified three broad strategies in crisis service as follows:[4]

- A parallel crisis service developed alongside existing referral systems;
- A crisis service as an integral part of the local mental health service with one entry point into the system; and
- A crisis service targeting a particular section of the mental health population. The service selects the time of referral and only accepts people who are judged to be appropriate for the methods employed by the team.

To date, little work has been done to compare the strengths of different models. Where crisis intervention services have been based on Caplan's theories using very focused short-term, therapeutic interventions (e.g., problem solving behavioral techniques), these interventions have usually excluded people with long-term needs by refusing referrals in which the individual is described as having a psychotic diagnosis. However, Caplan's theories may be useful in describing elements of services equally applicable for people with long-term needs.[5] The helping agency should be easy to contact and readily accessible. There must also be a willingness to work very intensively over a short period. Help should be time-limited, and long-term dependence should not be allowed to develop. The goal may be to return to the level of pre-crisis functioning rather than attempt more radical changes. It might be helpful to explore whether rigorous crisis intervention services are useful to people with long-term needs who are in the throes of a crisis.

The focus of much recent research has suggested that crisis services should either help prevent admission to a hospital or limit hospitalization to far shorter periods than would otherwise be the case. One of the longer established crisis intervention services serving a population of 350,000 found that the services admitted 30 percent fewer patients per 100,000 than the regional average and had a much lower proportion of compulsory admissions.

Research on the Sparkbrook home treatment program in Birmingham, which provides services to people with serious mental health problems, found that people who were admitted to the hospital and those involved in the Sparkbrook plan had similar diagnoses. Some of these home treatment patients had been treated in the hospital previously.

Issues concerning the form services should take and who should be providing them are still being debated. There are the questions of whether separate crisis support services should be provided for people with long-term needs, or whether people should use the traditional crisis services when their condition worsens. Two factors may be critical in helping to provide support to people with long-term needs during a crisis. First, it is essential to have some continuity between services to avoid having people readmitted to the acute service without receiving any other support. Second, a service has to offer a rapid, flexible response that is acceptable to those who are using it. In addition, there needs to be an effective mechanism such as case management to link all the services used by an individual. The role of the various professionals in crisis service and issues of multi-disciplinary intervention are also key elements of the debate.

Current Services

In Britain, 95 percent of mental health assistance is provided through the primary health care system by general practitioners and in some cases by counselors, nurses, or psychologists attached to general practitioners' practices. No doubt some crises are met without recourse to more specialized assistance. There have been other traditional means of providing a service in the community for people in a crisis. Some are supported by community psychiatric nurses, either attached to several general practitioners' practices or working as a district-based team. Others have been supported through psychiatric outpatient appointments or day hospital attendance.

Traditionally, crisis services have meant an inpatient admission, either to one of the large old Victorian institutions or to a psychiatric wing of a district general hospital (DGH). In the inner cities, these DGH services are becoming increasingly pressurized, with many compulsory admissions and few elective ones. Increasing levels of homelessness and the high incidence of serious mental health problems within this group are revealed in one inner city district, where 30 percent of the people admitted to the unit are homeless. Anecdotal reports suggest that the level of disturbance in the units has increased considerably. Given the limited facilities available in many areas, the community has also had to handle a far greater level of disturbance than previously.

People who use services also offer a number of criticisms. People go into hospitals for care, treatment, understanding, and safety. Service users suggest that they rarely find these desired elements of their hospitalization satisfactory and the only assistance available is generally medication. During the last 15 years, however, some more imaginative methods of service have been developed as pilot projects. In several areas, crisis services have been developed with psychiatrists working with a limited number of general practitioners' practices to provide a community service. Usually this service does not have direct access to inpatient care. One or two areas have established emergency walk-in psychiatric clinics providing access to services including inpatient ones, as required. The other main area of service development has been in community mental health centers.

Many of these community mental health centers identify provision of crisis service as part of their function. Where these services have been operating, many have focused on individuals who are anxious, depressed, or have less severe problems. Rarely do services go to those with serious mental health problems. This has been tackled in one or two community mental health centers by deliberately establishing services targeting people with these problems.

Possible Models For Future Service

The following section briefly describes three different models of service for people in crisis who have long-term mental health problems. Two of these services are already operating, and the third is in the detailed planning stage.

Camden Consortium: A Crisis House

In the Borough of Camden in 1986, Camden Consortium, a consumer organization, reviewed the services available to people with mental health problems. They identified a major need for crisis services available outside normal day center hours. The consortium's service review identified that the resources available at that time were either day centers closed evenings and weekends; emergency 24-hour support linked with hospital admission; or a Samaritan's telephone helpline not specifically designed for people in mental distress. There was a lack of overnight support in a crisis apart from a hospital.

The consortium identified three areas of need from the review:

- Readily available support, if necessary, on a 24-hour basis;
- A place to meet other people in the evenings or on weekends; and
- Occasional overnight care and accommodations outside of the hospital.

Initially, the consortium proposed a service based around a club. The club was intended to provide a good social environment and support for people who have had a history of mental illness. The facilities would include a snack bar, a member's telephone helpline available for use outside club hours, staff to provide support, and access to short-stay overnight accommodations. Funding was sought from various agencies including social services, health, and voluntary organizations. Unfortunately, with the financial situation worsening for all the welfare agencies, some amendments have had to be made to the proposals.

The consortium is now proposing that a staffed house be provided for people with mental health problems in a crisis. The house would operate quite differently from other existing services. A fundamental part of the philosophy is that people going to the house should be allowed to identify their own problems whether emotional or practical. A frequent experience of mental health service users is that professionals will identify problems quite differently from the way the patient does. The staff will be involved in helping provide the support the person needs and in ensuring that the person's life comes together while he or she is there. Planning for this service is now at a very advanced stage, and a job description is being circulated for the senior post. The service is being funded jointly by social services and the health authority.

Daily Living Programs At The Maudsley Hospital

The daily living program (DLP) was established in 1987 in an inner-city borough in London. A multi-cultural urban area was selected to replicate Test and Stein's community support programs, designed to provide considerable support to people with long-term mental health problems. People who presented themselves at a psychiatric emergency clinic at the Maudsley Hospital were randomly assigned to the DLP. A matched control group was established. After 18 months, there were 60 patients in each group; in early 1990 there were 92 people within the daily living program and 95 within the matched control group. The service is provided by seven nurses, a social worker, an occupational therapist, and a psychiatrist. The project was set up with four main aims: to provide continuity of care, case management, crisis intervention, and rehabilitation services. The service operates seven days a week, and a telephone service is available. Most people using the service have been diagnosed as having psychotic problems. About half of those using the service live alone.

The DLP has found that people need help with many areas of their lives—finances, housing, employment, legal matters, welfare benefits, and clinical assistance. People with serious mental health problems need consistent help over a long period of time. The team found that they were able to assist people with their clinical problems because those using the service trusted them after receiving help with the more practical difficulties, such as housing and finance.

There has been a considerable amount of research associated with the project. Some of this has focused on hospital admissions. A number of the DLP patients have been admitted to the hospital. After 18 months, 83 percent of the DLP patients had hospital stays; however, 50 percent had been in the hospital for three days or less. In the matched hospital group, 95 percent stayed in for more than three days and a number stayed in for more than two weeks. The DLP staff appear to be better able to identify who needs a longer period of stay in the hospital. The DLP group spent on average 16 days in the hospital, whereas the matched hospital group averaged 60 days. For people who had been diagnosed as suffering from a neurotic disorder, those within the DLP group averaged 1.9 days in the hospital, whereas the matched hospital group averaged 60 days. Although this figure should be used cautiously, so far, the cost of care for the DLP group would seem to be about 21 percent cheaper than hospital care.

Lewisham Mental Health Advice Center

The Lewisham Mental Health Advice Center (MHAC) was one of the first community mental health centers to be established in Britain. Initially, the center offered a walk-in service, accepting referrals from individuals in need of services, their families, or any agencies. Research on the MHAC, however, found that it was mainly assisting people with problems of living rather than with serious mental health problems. To remedy this imbalance, a crisis intervention team was established, staffed by a senior social worker, two community psychiatric nurses, and a psychiatric senior registrar. Two consultant psychiatrists responsible for the Lewisham community are also actively involved with the team and frequently visit. Four principle objectives have been identified for the service:

- To provide a rapid response to requests for psychiatric evaluation of disturbed and severely distressed clients.
- To institute and continue treatment of acute mental illness or emotional distress in the person's own home.
- To help members of the person's family understand the nature of the illness or distress and help them cope with their relative. To provide support and counseling for the person's family.
- Where treatment at home is inappropriate, to make alternative arrangements for care including hospital admission, if necessary.

The crisis intervention team operates on an open referral basis. Initial assessments are performed by two members of the team working together, usually in the person's home. They are usually undertaken on the same day that the referral is received. Cases are managed by a key worker, discussed regularly, and kept open until the satisfactory resolution of the crisis which may necessitate admission. There are usually between three and seven referrals received each week and the team is likely to be carrying a caseload of around 20–30 clients. Research has indicated that the team's clients are more likely to be younger, male, Afro-Caribbeans suffering from schizophrenia, major affective disorders, or other serious mental illnesses.

To provide a comprehensive service, a continuing care team was also established at the Mental Health Advisory Center. The team is oriented towards rehabilitation and providing continuing practical support to people with long-term mental health problems. Theoretically, there is a distinction between the intervention team and the continuing care element of the service. In practice people with long-term needs may continue to be supported by workers from the crisis intervention team. Once people have developed a relationship, they may be reluctant to pass over the case to someone else.

In conclusion, fundamental questions about crisis services for people with long-term needs deserve further exploration. There are several innovative services operating in different parts of the country. These need to be evaluated, information on them disseminated more widely, and attempts made to identify the circumstances that may best suit a particular model. Some key factors can be identified for these services to be successful. First, services need to be integrated with existing mental health provisions in the area. They also need to target people with long-term needs and be provided in a way that can both reach people with serious mental health problems and be acceptable to them.

As far as the content of the service is concerned, a range of services has to be offered from clinical assessment, counseling, and therapeutic interventions to very practical forms of assistance. The staff group providing the services will need to have relevant skills and professional backgrounds to draw upon. In many places, this will mean extending the existing repertoire of skills for helping people in a crisis beyond simply offering medication to more imaginative solutions, including continued practical assistance in the client's home.

Notes

1. G. Caplan, *Principles of Preventive Psychiatry*, (New York: Basic Books, 1964).
2. T. Farewell, "Crisis Intervention," *Nursing Mirror* (September 2), 69–70, 1967.
3. L. Ratna, "The Practice of Psychiatric Crisis Intervention," (Napsbury Hospital League of Friends, 1978).
4. S. Newton, "Organizational Models for Crisis Intervention," Crisis Intervention Information Pack, *Good Practices in Mental Health* (London, 1986).
5. G. Waldron, "Crisis Intervention—A Persistent Theme," Crisis Intervention Information Pack, Good Practices in Mental Health, (London, 1986).

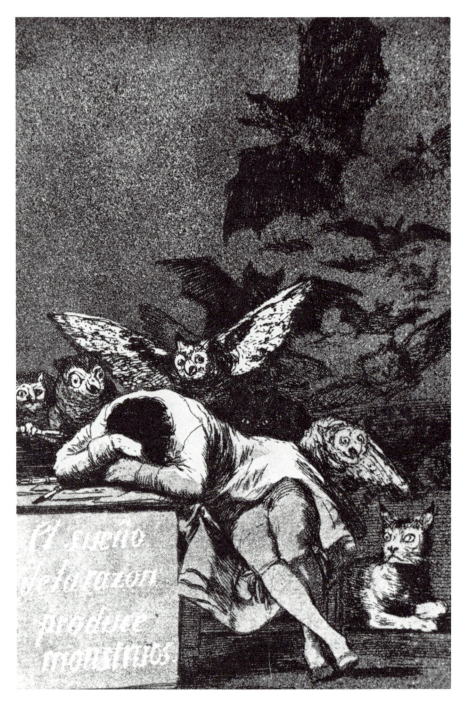

The Sleep of Reason Produces Monsters. Etching and aquatint ca. 1797. Courtesy of The Bettmann Archive.

❧ CASE MANAGEMENT

By Yvonne Christie

The Griffiths report (1988) looked at the importance of collaboration among the health authority, local authority, and the voluntary sector to deliver good quality services for people with long-term needs. The report highlighted a gap in the existing system of mental health services delivery. This is the need to have a designated person planning individual care packages and drawing upon the full range of community services to help people live ordinary lives. This individual would also ensure the best use of resources and prevent duplication of efforts by various service providers.

The government formalized this notion in the white paper, "Caring for People." It states that no one who is a patient of a consultant psychiatrist should be discharged from a psychiatric hospital without a care plan. The report notes that when an individual's needs are complex or a certain level of resources is involved, then a case manager should be appointed to assess and review the person's needs and ensure effective management of resources.

The case manager could be employed by the local authority, but this is not always necessary. Indeed, nurses may also be as well-suited to the role as may others. From our experience of case management models in the United Kingdom, some of the steps for effective case management should include the following:

- Identification of people in need (including open access systems for referral);
- Assessment of care needs;
- Planning and securing the delivery of care;
- Monitoring the quality of care provided; and
- Review of client needs.

It is not the role of case managers to actually deliver the services involved in an individual's care plan, but rather to ensure that other workers are delivering the services agreed upon in the plan and to provide a realistic time-span for achieving goals and reviewing progress. If a person is to be a full participant in the community, then a range of service providers, friends, and volunteers will need to be involved. The white paper does not state that case managers should be the purse holders, although the case management process should be linked with the budgeting and finance system to ensure a care plan can be implemented with available resources.

Case management provides the opportunity to view people as individuals, and to assess their health and social needs in a comprehensive manner. It also creates the opportunity for an imaginative response to peoples' needs which may move beyond the traditional service responses. This approach is invaluable, especially when working with people from minority racial groups. Presently, such people passing through our mental health system feel that their needs are inadequately addressed—if at all. Many mental health workers would agree with this and welcome case management as a process that may prove helpful in delivering an ethnically-sensitive service. The case manager will have to involve the caregiver or family member as well as the user in determining individual plans. Relevant local resources will have to be used, and experienced members of the community will be called upon to ensure the delivery of the approved package of care. However, the authorities still need to greatly improve their training and their communication networks to ensure that they have an understanding of what is appropriate and available for a person from a different race or culture.

Contracts for care should be used innovatively. Agencies experienced in working with minority racial populations should be fully utilized. The government has stated that the use of the voluntary sector and the promotion of a mixed economy of care will increase the choices available to users. However, it remains to be seen whether the needs of minority racial populations and others with long-term problems are part of the plan from the beginning, or are tacked on at the end of community care plans and thus excluded from real participation in the process.

Gateshead Case Management Service

The Gateshead Council has organized a scheme for elderly people. The population of Gateshead is spread across a large rural area with some elderly people living in remote locations where they are unable to have gas service to their homes. This community care scheme began eight years ago, and its aim is to help vulnerable elderly people remain at home. It works with the help of volunteers who are engaged on a contractual basis.

The senior social worker constructs a budget for the year and devises packages of care for individuals. The eligibility criteria for the project are that the person must be over pensionable age and must be at the stage of referral for residential services. Referrals can be made through social services, general practitioners, family members, friends, or directly by clients. The social worker assesses and plans packages of care for the clients and also offers support for the volunteers who deliver the home-based services. To date, volunteers are recruited through local networks, and they are given ongoing training. An issue of concern for the Gateshead project is how to utilize the volunteers when their services in a particular area are no longer required. To keep training people and then laying them off is a continuing problem.

With each elderly person referred to the project, the social worker plans his/her budget. This procedure becomes much easier as prices are worked out for equipment, expenses, training of volunteers, and other costs. Out of this budget, the social worker also plans short-term respite for the client's caregiver. However, this project has run into difficulties with a change in line management. The new director of social services is not as supportive of the scheme and, because of the project's lack of independence from the local authority, there is a threat of it being discontinued.

A case manager with this type of project can work with 20–25 cases, but this has serious resource implications if all eligible people are to be offered the service. The white paper states that everyone leaving the hospital, as well as people with special needs, should have a case manager (legislation on this will be enforced starting in 1991). It is not yet known whether the resources will be made available to undertake this task.

Choice Project

The Choice Project exemplifies an independent case management service in operation. It is funded through charity donations and funding from both health and social services, thereby giving it independent status. To date, the project has served people with physical disabilities. Referrals are either made directly from hospitals or through friends, families, or social workers. The project is structured on the belief that people with disabilities have the same rights as other human beings, and the project workers draw upon a whole range of community services to enable people to take charge of their own lives as much as possible. The workers believe in giving individuals full involvement in their packages of care regardless of the severity of the disabilities. It is usually this important aspect of the planning for a person's care package that is missing, leading, in turn, to individuals having a service that does not meet their needs.

The present workers have organized a procedure to ensure that case management works for the user. They feel that a case manager should be able to do the following:

- Coordinate an assessment of need—i.e., a person's medical, social, and financial situation;
- Clarify which other professionals are involved with their client and which professionals to draw experience from;
- Analyze information, agree on goals with their clients, identify blocks to progress, and help service providers to review their services and highlight gaps;
- Build up relationships with service providers by negotiating across agencies and interagency boundaries;
- Work creatively and use resources in an imaginative way;
- Act as a support or formal representative at tribunals or appeals; and

- Understand and learn about community resources, national services, the local council, and legal procedures, and be informed about the consumer movement.

Some of the personal attributes the workers have had to develop are persistence, persuasiveness, approachability by the public, confidence, and friendliness. In order to assess whether or not their service is working, the staff have regular reviews where they record and collate information on the needs of users. This information is important for policymaking and planning processes which may include joint-care planning teams, local consumer groups, disability and pressure groups, public awareness initiatives, and other activities.

It will be interesting to see how the role of case manager develops in this country, whether the workers involved will be a separate and independent group of people as in the Choice Project or whether posts will be revamped from existing social worker positions. If the latter occurs, we may lose a valuable opportunity to offer a truly individualized service to people in need.

∼ RESETTLEMENT FROM HOSPITAL*

By Helen Smith

The implementation of community-based mental health services in Great Britain is a dreadfully slow process. The policy is more than 30 years old, allowing enough time to have sorted out the fundamental issues of structural change, to have developed the range of community services and facilities people need, and to have at least reduced reliance on long-stay hospital provision. Despite general acceptance of the ideas of community care and evidence of an accelerating pace of change, the practice is patchy and woefully inadequate.

The Management Of Change

Community care is about the management of change on a grand scale. It is not simply about dealing with marginal changes within a well-developed service structure but about fundamentally redesigning care and support systems. At strategic decision-making levels, there are political and financial pressures to contend with. At the point of service delivery, the reasons for change can be taken as implied criticism of professional competence and practice. Users, relatives, and the general public have been alarmed by the prospect of change.

Resettlement of people from the hospital is one part of a wider change in the provision of mental health services. Districts and local authorities have undertaken the planning of comprehensive services by doing the following:

- Stating the principles underlying the process of development based on service users' needs;
- Formulating ways to meet those needs;
- Consulting with others in the system;
- Reformulating plans in the light of comments;
- Gaining support, approval, and finance for plans; and
- Continually refining plans in the light of experience.

*Adapted from D. Braisby, R. Echlin, S. Hill, and H. Smith. *Changing Futures: Housing and Support Services for People Discharged from Psychiatric Hospitals* (London: King Edward's Hospital Fund, 1988).

Plans should not be cast in stone. At present, plans are discussed with many people but rarely those for whom the service is designed. Once financial resources are allocated to specific schemes within a plan, it is often difficult to change them. This is precisely what needs to happen in order to find better ways to achieve the service aims, especially if the original design is neither wanted nor needed by service users. A total resource approach to planning has been emphasized by the department of health in relation to the role of the joint consultative committees (JCCs) in joint planning. This has helped stimulate fresh perspectives and new partnerships with those traditionally excluded from the planning process. Managers of current statutory and voluntary services have found ways to pool their knowledge and examine familiar resources and local problems from different perspectives. Encouraging staff and the people they serve to participate in the planning and implementation of a new service fosters commitment.

The resettlement of people from a large hospital to much smaller services in local communities poses many difficult questions concerning personnel policies, managerial style, and funding mechanisms—especially in projects utilizing multidisciplinary teams. Although many such projects are working successfully, there is not yet sufficient experience out of which to develop any particular structural model. One approach is the new task-oriented local voluntary agency set up as a means of bringing together service providers, additional resources, and specific expertise. For example, several London authorities are setting up consortia of local housing, health, social services, and voluntary agencies within the framework of charitable companies. Their constitutions can provide for equal partnership through representatives of the constituent member organizations. Although the principal aim is usually the finance, development, and subsequent management of housing, the provision of care and related support can also be arranged and coordinated either directly by the consortium or through the respective constituent members.

The resettlement of people in most districts is being phased in over several years. Some districts are using a project-based approach which utilizes the accumulated experience of resettling people from long-stay hospitals. Although the nature, range, and scope of developed services and facilities varies considerably, they have several things in common including delays in implementation.

The main advantage of the project-based approach is that the local experience of developing new projects can be useful in future projects. In other words, the pioneering, trail-blazing project prepares the way for subsequent projects. The negotiation of access to people living in hospital wards, deciding who will move to new facilities, developing new care delivery and management systems, scheduling capital and revenue funding, and the general acceptance of community projects become easier the second and third time around. Problems may still occur in the recruitment, redeployment, training, and retention of staff. There may also be delays in building and adapting programs, obtaining planning consents, and arranging adequate long-term financing; but at least a more realistic appraisal of the development process is being incorporated into future implementation plans.

Certainly these pioneering projects are highlighting inadequacies in the system as a whole. However, despite the patchiness of implementation nationally, it is clear that where there is local commitment to change, these difficulties can generally be overcome.

Resettlement Services in the Hospital

The decision to close a hospital is a commitment to carry through a complete move of all patients. We are just now gaining experience on how to develop service options for people based on more explicit knowledge of their needs and wishes. The initial problems center around accommodations. Resettlement teams seek out what individual choices there are, so that at the outset, planners will know they are on the right track. Housing and other facilities often take a long time to obtain, and staff can experience a frustrating delay between availability and active preparation for discharge.

As a general rule of good practice, some project directors have found it useful to observe the "least moves" principle which avoids moving people from ward to ward prior to community discharge. This enables them to move directly to their most desired living environment. Also, taking social networks into account within the hospital, some people may want to live with friends who are not residents in designated closure wards. Thus, for people not yet ready to make a decision to move out, short-term bed spaces may become available.

Often those with mental health difficulties have problems developing or holding onto their social networks. People who have lived in a psychiatric hospital for a long time will have particular difficulties moving into the community unless staff recognize the importance of existing social networks in the hospital. Hospital friendships often cross boundaries of ward, age, or disability, while new contacts in the community may follow social limitations.

In some resettlement services, project contact teams identify individuals and find out what additional resources and services they need. This information is relayed to service providers. Good contact teams are mainly comprised of resettlement staff who provide continuity between hospital and community. A major part of their role is to help people prepare for a new life and to give continued support in the community. Whether team members are drawn from a number of different agencies or are specially recruited depends on local considerations.

The first step for project contact teams is to establish a presence in a chosen ward and get people used to the idea of change. Experience suggests that each member of a contact team can eventually manage an active workload of three to six people, depending on the range of needs. Following a decision to move, someone may need full-time attention for at least three months prior to discharge. A full-time multidisciplinary team of six staff gathering information directly from the people themselves, explaining their role, and helping to prepare individuals for discharge can start resettling a ward within four to six months from first contact.

The ward should close completely in about 18 months, provided housing and support services become available.

The key factors affecting the way contact teams organize their work are the number of staff and wards involved, the time scale, and the objectives. A typical resettlement project deals with 15 housing units and a total of 30 bed spaces. The plan is to find housing for five people each month in three monthly intervals allowing serial resettlement. In theory, once the first houses are ready, the contact team of six have 18 months to resettle 30 people, splitting their time between hospital and community. In practice, the development process is uncertain because buildings are not always available. Once houses are ready to hand over, resettlement must occur quickly to meet charges for rent and so on.

Furthermore, as people are resettled, more staff are added for support. Following the principle of continuity of care, contact team members begin to develop individual plans in the hospital and become care coordinators in the new service, working directly with other care workers and the people who are resettled. How many other care workers are needed will depend on a range of factors peculiar to each project. In the example cited, at least six more will be needed. Managers must be able to respond quickly to the need to bring in extra staff as necessary.

Some teams have found it useful, particularly when contact teams from different facilities are working in the same ward, to set up a forum for exchanging information on a regular basis. In their experience, the forum should be established as soon as contact teams start negotiating access to the wards. Indeed, such negotiation should take place through that forum. A service provider's forum would include hospital staff, the resettlement team, management, and other interested parties such as voluntary organizations and users. It would have flexible membership in order to involve different people in the different stages of identification, assessment, and preparation of people for transfer to new facilities.

In some places user-only forums have also been developed with initial staff support. The aim is to enable users to discuss the changes, give their opinions on plans presented to them, and to elect representatives to work on planning teams, service provider forums, and other activities.

The getting-to-know-you process is one approach to developing relationships between individuals and resettlement workers. The process also ideally lends itself to the development of an individual plan (IP) which is a statement of care and support strategies. IPs should include attainable goals which will gradually increase confidence, self-esteem, and a sense of life control. As a working document, the plan should reflect all relevant views and be reviewed regularly. The subject of the plan also must freely agree to its content.

The utilization of external contact teams as agents of resettlement from hospitals and eventually as care coordinators or key workers in the new service will ensure continuity of care. It is probably best that hospital staff do not immediately move out with their residents. The step from "patients to people" is an important one and staff will need time and training to adapt to new ways of working. However, given further training, ward staff who have seen their wards close in the way described will have picked up enough information to assist in future ward closures.

One of the primary tasks in developing community-based resettlement services is to clearly identify and provide a range of housing options. There are a number of ways that this can be done.

Housing could be provided directly according to need. This would require an assessment of the people leaving the hospital and moving into the district. Given that it takes time for resettlement workers to get to know individuals and help them reach an informed choice on housing, this approach may not prove feasible. For workers to obtain information on housing from all people returning to a district would probably require two or three years.

An alternative approach is to make assumptions about the range of housing needs. Tower Hamlets Mental Health and Housing Working Party undertook a survey of need for accommodation and support services for a representative sample of people who were long-term users of the mental health services. They compiled a register of long-stay inpatients, frequent admissions, and clinic and day center attenders. They also gathered information through questionnaires completed by staff and interviews with users and staff. The information was compiled and placed on a scale measuring dependence, activity, effects of current symptoms, and degree of isolation/inactivity. The survey yielded valuable information and enabled the working party to predict fairly accurately the accommodation needs for the entire district.

This type of survey could be adapted for use with people in the hospital. Getting to know a sample of service users in depth may provide sufficient information to predict overall housing needs. Hospital assessment methods are also useful measures, but the resettlement workers should be wary of relying only on hospital-based information. Staff from wards designated for closure may not be the most appropriate people to do individual assessments. To ensure a fresh look at each person, unaffected by preconceptions of their abilities, a new group of staff should coordinate individual assessments and make predictions on housing needs. In practice, this will most probably be the resettlement or contact team.

Whatever the predictions of housing needs, a range of options will be made available. These will include staffed homes, multi-occupancy homes, single flats, adult fostering, respite care provision, and other options. Clearly, liaisons with the local authority, housing associations, and/or voluntary organizations are essential at the earliest planning stages.

During these early stages, crisis services and respite care facilities will have to be established for the first discharges from hospitals. This will be a time of high stress and anxiety for people, requiring skilled, sensitive support to ensure they do not end up in a psychiatric admission ward.

In shared living arrangements, people do not always get along with each other and it may be that alternative arrangements will have to be made within a few months following discharge. The use of admission wards in such circumstances would be entirely inappropriate. Temporary alternative accommodation pending a more long-term solution may be essential to prevent a drama from becoming a crisis that consumes staff resources and causes considerable distress to those involved. Such a facility may help to prevent the demoralization that can occur if a person or placement appears to have failed. Obviously, the contact team will be working hard with people during these first months, but other specialist crisis services should be available. Indeed, crisis teams will form an integral part of a community-based service.

Resettlement In Practice

In summary, the resettlement program devised by MIND in Waltham Forest found that it was eight months from the initial contact with ward staff before the first house (2x2 bed flats) was resettled and 15 months before 13 people were finally resettled in four houses. The initial contact team of three grew to a direct-care team of six. The average client age was 55. Ranging from 35 to 68 years old, this group had accumulated 27 years of contact with psychiatric services, mostly in institutional care. Staff do not live in the resettlement houses.

Firm decisions about household composition were not made until three months before a move. Subsequently this was considered an absolute minimum of time for staff to get acquainted with, formally assess, and help prepare people for moving. Some people were quite definite about household partners while others needed help with deciding the household composition.

For all concerned, relationships were developed mostly through practical tasks such as cooking, choosing furniture and house color schemes, and generally finding out about the local area. Although skills were acquired and practiced before the move, the period was characteristically one of psychological preparation. The most effective learning situation would be the new environment, which is where staff resources were most concentrated.

Resettlement Work In The Community

Good, permanent accommodation is the cornerstone of community care, but there are many other components. For instance, people leaving long-stay psychiatric hospitals need help with structuring their day. They also need support in using ordinary community facilities such as shops, cafes, schools, and sport and leisure accommodations which offer opportunities to mix with others in the community. In order to achieve this level of integration, people moving back to the community need to have a system of personal support set up for them, probably for the rest of their lives.

Although community care has been discussed for the last 30 years, we are only now starting to know how to develop flexible, responsive support services needed to maintain people with long-term mental illness in the community. There has been greater momentum behind the development of community mental health teams and centers where the emphasis is on acute care, rather than on people with long-term problems. Community care is developing in such a way that it is too easy for the needs and interests of those with the most severe disabilities to be overlooked.

In any support system, there is an inherent danger that the level of support will smother initiative and prevent people from taking control over their lives. Support staff are in the challenging position of having to meet genuine needs but, at the same time, encourage initiative and positive risk-taking. Institutionalized services encouraged dependence; therefore, in order to avoid recreating the same problems in a new service, support should be provided flexibly, taking individual progress into account. Experience is showing that people should not be prevented from attempting new tasks or having new experiences because of predetermined assumptions about their capacity for change and growth. Indeed, there are now many success stories which no one ever thought possible.

People with severe psychological disabilities are no different from the rest of us in their need for a social network to support them in a neighborhood or community. Unfortunately, their disabilities are often expressed in such a way that they have difficulty maintaining such networks. Good resettlement projects have made it a major service aim to maintain or extend people's social networks. Resettlement and other care staff have applied appropriate, nonintrusive ways of building networks. It is generally thought that those who have severe mental health problems are loners who prefer not to have contact with other people. In fact, their lives are often devoid of the shared experiences which make social contact possible and natural for most people. They may have lost touch with their past, but trips to see family and old friends help restore a sense of continuity in time and place.

Experience indicates that most of the social and practical skills that people need to acquire, apart from basic safety skills, are best learned in the environment in which they will be used rather than in the hospital prior to discharge. This is different from the ladder model of rehabilitation, which prepares people for increasingly independent stages of living to which they must graduate. The staff needs to provide support in daily living skills, such as self-care, housework, shopping, and budgeting. Apart from tasks centered around running a home, the person may also need help in interacting with members of the community at various times while using public transportation to visit shops, cafes, and other ordinary community facilities. A great deal of help may be needed at first, but the level of support can be gradually reduced as people become more skilled.

The need to teach skills in real environments demands flexibility from staff members. They need to be prepared to work in different settings, in a person's home or elsewhere in the community, and to withdraw or increase support as needed. They also need negotiation skills to meet an individual's needs and wishes in ordinary community settings.

One example of good practice in flexible support is the work of the Peter Bedford Trust, a voluntary organization which provides housing and employment for over 100 people with institutional backgrounds. The Trust employs a team of three full-time support workers who combine traditional housing management functions with support work. They assist individuals with everyday tasks and also encourage the tenants to carry these out for themselves. Help is provided with household cleaning, personal hygiene, financial advice, education, and liaison with mental health services. Most of the tenants take part in the Trust's work schemes during the day. The level of support varies according to individual needs and ranges from weekly contact for rent collection to regular visits or weekend stays with someone who is ill. A small number of tenants who lack basic living skills do not go out to work and three additional part-time workers provide intensive training for these people in their own homes. An education and training officer has been appointed to develop leisure and educational opportunities for the tenants in nonsegregated community settings. This officer's work also includes the design of training programs for the part-time support workers. In addition, institutional trainers are educated in the types of skills that people discharged from long-stay hospitals need in the community.

In spite of the existence of a long-term support system, service users may require intensive support during crises and may even need to move out of their homes for a while. Possible forms of assistance must be considered at the development stage of any project. Where there are no resident staff, an emergency service should be in place which can be quickly activated if a tenant becomes acutely distressed. For example, the Forest Community Project, run by Waltham Forest MIND, has installed an expensive, but effective, mobile telephone system so that the duty worker is on call should the need arise.

Some local mental health services have found ways of providing intensive support over a short period. For example, the North Derbyshire Mental Health Services Project has a peripatetic rehabilitation team that is able to provide 24-hour care in a tenant's home if necessary. The project has also allocated a small budget to its network of self-help support groups so that if one member is acutely distressed, practical help and support can be provided quickly.

Earning power is a problem for people on long-term benefits who are poor and severely restricted in the number of opportunities they have for ordinary social activities. The financial arrangements surrounding the transfer from hospital to community and for handling a tenant's income afterwards can be particularly devaluing. Furnishing a home to a high standard and buying new clothes are important to enhancing self image, yet problems in getting the money through the Social Fund (a grant payable to individuals who lack basic amenities) for such essential items often causes the person to feel even more devalued. People need particularly sensitive support, therefore, in learning how to budget and control their own finances.

Housing management is another basic task in a residential service and usually consists of arranging leases, collecting the rent, and advising the resident on repairs and maintenance. Where local authority housing is used, these tasks are normally carried out by a housing worker, and direct care and support is provided by social services. A small voluntary organization supporting three or four people in a housing association property may employ one worker to carry out both management and support tasks. Some perceive a conflict between representing the landlord and providing care and support to the tenant. There is much disagreement among service providers about whether one task interferes with the other. Housing management and counseling appear to be quite separate functions. However, those who favor the one-worker arrangement argue that housing staff are regularly drawn into tenants' personal problems and that their friendly advice may be more helpful than counseling from an official source.

People resettled in the community also need some meaningful way to occupy their time. Although work is the most valued form of occupation, unemployment rates make it necessary to provide alternatives. In addition, most ordinary housing schemes are financed in such a way that even though employed, people still could not afford to pay the charges. Differential charges can be made for people who work, but there is no incentive for agencies to find work for their tenants.

Organizing The Support Service

Community mental health teams are being developed to do some of the necessary support work. On the whole, however, they are showing a greater interest in acute care than in working with people with long-term problems. Existing primary care services which include general practitioners, community psychiatric nurses, and social services also have a role to play. Two basic approaches to long-term care are evolving.

In the first approach, an independent worker or team of workers provides care and support to tenants in one or more houses dispersed over a small locality. There are links with health and social services staff who may be called in to provide emergency care if needed. This model is usually chosen by voluntary organizations which develop housing projects in conjunction with housing associations. If a voluntary agency has a single house supported by one worker, there may be problems in providing coverage for holidays or sick leave. The advantage of a team is that the workers can get to know all the tenants so that individuals do not experience a loss of continuity of care if their regular worker is absent. Training and supervision is also easier to arrange for a team than for individuals.

Because of the lack of training opportunities elsewhere, the team usually arranges its own training program. An individual worker does not have the resources to do this. The variety of skills within a generic team can also potentially provide richer experiences for tenants, including interpersonal skills.

Such an approach is being developed by Waltham Forest MIND. Set up as a pilot project in supported housing service, the Forest Community Project is using a team of generic workers to provide care and support to people with a long history of psychiatric disabilities who now live in a small number of houses scattered throughout one neighborhood. Most members of the team are mental health professionals. Outside professional services are arranged as needed. The team is also developing a community center which will provide an office base for the staff and a social facility, including a snack bar, for the tenants and local community.

The second approach involves a team of care workers attached to a community mental health team (CMHT) which provides long-term support to tenants in a dispersed network of houses. Members of the CMHT also carry out regular work with the tenants and provide emergency care. There are a number of variations of this model. Some health authorities have set up CMHTs specifically to provide primary and acute care rather than support or rehabilitation services. In these cases, there may be plans to develop separate support teams at a later stage. There are advantages and disadvantages to linking the community mental health and community support teams. The support staff may be tempted to work with people whose progress is more immediately rewarding rather than concentrate their efforts on people with long-term needs. However, people with relatively minor problems can benefit from contact with those who have long-term needs and vice versa. Access to a primary care team also means that people with long-term needs are given the same opportunities for change and growth as other people.

In the London borough of Camden, a team of domiciliary care workers is being established for a small group of tenants who have recently been discharged from a long-stay psychiatric hospital. The care workers will not necessarily be qualified in mental health work, but will receive appropriate training. This team is attached to a multidisciplinary community mental health team which will provide services to all mental health facilities within a given geographical area. Both care workers and professionals will be involved in direct work with tenants. In addition to providing support to people who have left the hospital, the support staff will also provide a service to people with severe mental health problems who have largely remained living in their own homes. Where people are being cared for by relatives, these caregivers will also be given counseling and other supportive services.

A great deal of development work has gone into building teams in which staff from different disciplines and backgrounds can work well together. However, most teams agree that particular attention needs to be paid to information systems so that individual service users do not get lost in the complex service system. There are few good computerized systems in this country and the issue of case tracking through computerized registers is just now gaining in priority.

Bricks And Mortar

In Great Britain we are hopefully moving from a buildings-based service to a network of human services; yet we must still consider new ways of providing housing and day care facilities. The crux of the problem with buildings is the way they are used and whether they allow integration or promote institutionalization and restriction. It can be argued that no building inherently promotes institutionalization, but the larger the building and the more people living there, the greater the degree of internal organizational control required. There is less flexibility and more allowance for individual differences in large buildings. A ward or hostel of 24 people will generally function as a homogeneous unit. In contrast, a number of one- to four-bed flats and houses can still be managed as a unit and this range allows for individual differences in expression of personal style and choice. Small-scale housing accommodations also encourage a more individualized approach from direct care staff.

From research we know about the kind of housing that people discharged from the hospital prefer to live in. In a recent study carried out in two London boroughs, a majority of those interviewed said that they wanted to live in independent, permanent accommodations.[1] Some conclusions about preferred types of housing can also be drawn from the experiences that the mentally ill have in existing types of specialist housing. How would any of us feel about living in a large hostel that stood out from the surrounding neighborhood or in a house with eight or nine other ex-patients, none of whom has anything to do during the day? No one values living in housing which is institutional in appearance or in practice.

Ordinary housing has been used to provide a small-scale network service which can provide both accommodation and support services. Within these services, there is a variety of housing which can be adapted to meet individual needs. Most people have chosen to live either by themselves or with one or two other people. Occasionally four-bedroom houses are provided by these services but, on the whole, a better quality of life has been achieved in smaller groups.

From the accumulated experiences of these projects, three other major considerations, apart from size, have emerged in developing good practice in ordinary housing.

First, the housing should be dispersed so that there is no risk of creating small communities or "ghettos" of mentally ill people. Another consideration is the proximity of housing or day facilities for other groups, such as those with mental or physical handicaps. Grouping such people together, because they are so devalued by society, will draw attention to them and hinder their integration into the local community. To prevent several sites from being developed in the same neighborhood, there needs to be good cooperation and communication among the various agencies involved. A local authority planning or housing department could possibly play a coordinating role in gathering information about housing developments for people with various disabilities in order to prevent grouping them together.

Ideally, there should not be more than one house on each street, although this would depend on other factors such as the length of the street or availability of housing. The properties should be spread out over a small locality, perhaps two miles in radius, and be within walking distance of each other. This would allow staff to work easily since it cannot be assumed that each worker has a car. Each house or flat should have on-street parking close by to allow ease of access.

Second, the properties should be close to shops and all the other ordinary community facilities. They should be within easy reach of the discharged patient's workplace or the community center that the resident might use during the day. Proximity to public transportation routes is also an important consideration because it is easy for people with mental illness to become isolated on large run-down housing estates.

In rural areas it may not be possible to locate housing within a small neighborhood where all of an individual's needs can be met. The housing network may be more widely dispersed and development workers may have to think of imaginative ways of meeting day care needs on an outreach basis. The North Derbyshire Mental Health Services Project, based in Chesterfield, has overcome some of the problems of covering a large rural area by developing self-help support groups in the outlying market towns of the Peak District. A project worker provides back-up to each group but they are essentially self-governing.

Third, since noise is a well-known cause of stress, properties should be on quiet streets where there is no continuous or intermittent noise from road or rail traffic, factories, or schools. Because it is not always possible to meet this requirement in cities, various kinds of sound insulation, such as double glazing, should be considered. In addition to reducing noise from outside, some attention should be paid to creating a quiet environment within the house. Insulation between floors is essential to cut down noise from upstairs flats, for example.

In conclusion, ordinary housing has to be converted by careful design to provide a variety of accommodations to suit individual needs. Normally tenants have their own rooms with a shared sitting room. A spare room for overnight visitors is sometimes provided. Some tenants have exclusive use of facilities such as kitchens and bathrooms. Sharing intensively-used facilities is a potential source of conflict, but careful design can overcome some of these problems. For example, a three-bedroom house can be converted to provide two partially self-contained units for one or two people with a shared sitting room. In a three-bedroom house, the residents might share all the facilities. Decisions about design have to be made with adequate knowledge of an individual's wishes, needs, and abilities.

Ordinary housing has been used to provide permanent homes for people discharged from long-stay hospitals. However, most people move from time to time, and people with mental illnesses are no exception. They may wish to change flatmates or, with increasing age, may wish to move to a ground-floor flat closer to shops. The housing network, therefore, has to budget for a few vacancies at any one time so that some movement among properties can take place. It is important to distinguish between a freely-made decision to move and the ladder model of rehabilitation where people are pushed to move from stepping-stone villas to half-way houses to rehabilitation hostels and finally to independent housing. People should not move solely because their needs for staff support have increased; services should always be brought to the person where possible. People should have to move out of their own home only if the service they need cannot be provided there. They should stay away for as short a time as possible and then return home.

Housing Availability

Ordinary housing is the ideal, but in practice, people on low incomes or benefits have a restricted choice of housing. Currently, people leaving the hospital have the following choices: to return to their own or their family's home; to move into ordinary rented accommodations run by local authority or housing associations; to stay in specialist accommodations, such as hostels or group homes, perhaps for a limited period; or to use emergency accommodations.

Most ordinary housing schemes have made use of local authority's rented accommodations or have developed special projects in conjunction with housing associations. The type of housing used and the way it is financed depends very much on local factors, such as relationships between the statutory bodies and voluntary organizations.

Some housing schemes have been successful in making extensive use of public sector housing. Under the Housing (Homeless Persons) Act of 1977, local authorities have a duty to rehouse people deemed vulnerable, which includes people with mental illnesses. However, not all local authorities will accept people as being homeless while they are still in the hospital. Some housing departments operate a quota system so that priority can be given to people with mental illnesses. Where local authority housing is used, it is important to involve housing department staff at an early stage so that they are aware of the needs of the people they are being asked to rehouse. Local authorities are an increasingly important source of housing for people with mental illnesses, but it is still unusual for housing departments to be represented on joint planning teams (JPTs). It is especially important to involve them in housing sub-groups of JPTs or in community-based resettlement planning groups.

Some resettlement teams have worked with housing staff to make them aware of the process of social devaluation and the need to counteract it by choosing the most socially-valued housing option. It may be tempting for housing departments to allocate hard-to-rent accommodations, but they need to be aware that people leaving psychiatric hospitals have a greater need for high-quality accommodations than other people. People with mental illnesses should not be allocated housing which will lead to a vicious circle of stress, breakdown, and readmission to the hospital. Some housing departments now refer to hard-to-rent tower blocks as vertical sheltered accommodations. It is up to care providers to ensure that housing authorities have adequate information about the needs of people with severe disabilities, so that this type of housing is not allocated.

Similarly, people with mental illnesses may need greater protection from crime than other people. People with disabilities, whether psychological or physical, are particularly vulnerable to become crime victims, so housing in areas with high rates of vandalism and crime should never be allocated to them.

Many housing associations are now interested in developing special projects for people leaving psychiatric care. Joint financing and, more recently, housing association grants have made it possible for health authorities to supply part or all the funds for a housing association to purchase a house. Health authorities can also provide add-on revenue contributions. The arrangements for financing special housing are complex. Since housing associations have expertise in the acquisition and management of property but lack knowledge of mental health services, they are anxious to work with statutory or voluntary agencies that know more about the needs of people with mental illnesses. The usual arrangement is that housing associations provide the buildings in partnership with a statutory or voluntary agency, which then acts as the managing agent of the property and provides care and support to the tenants.

In order to overcome some of the problems of shared responsibilities, some London housing associations have initiated the notion of the consortium. Technically, consortia could also employ and manage community care staff, but this function is not yet well-developed.

For some people, a family sponsorship arrangement may provide the most suitable form of accommodation. Some local authorities operate adult care schemes which enable them to match individuals with suitable careers. Even people with severe disabilities can be resettled in this way.

Lodging for people with mental illnesses has acquired a bad name and has sometimes become associated with seaside boarding houses and profiteering landlords. Little or no care is provided and individuals are quietly forgotten. However, for some groups of people such as single, older men, lodging in someone else's home is a normal and socially accepted type of accommodation. There is no reason why the staff in a housing network should not support one or two people in such lodgings if this were thought to be the most appropriate accommodation for them. The London Borough of Camden, as part of its adult care scheme, has recruited landladies who are prepared to offer accommodations to people with mental health problems. Although the borough has pioneered this type of adult care scheme, the disadvantage is that people with mental illnesses are often actually placed outside the borough and consequently lose touch with their normal social networks. Landladies need to be given training in providing care to people who have been institutionalized and need to know that professional support can be summoned whenever they need it.

Family sponsorship and lodgings seem to work best in rural areas, perhaps because there is a higher degree of community integration. In some places, landladies are able to join a support group so that they can meet to exchange information and discuss problems.

Ordinary Housing In Practice

Although it is possible to describe the kind of housing that is wanted, the road to establishing people in ordinary housing is paved with rules and regulations, which may be in conflict with the principles outlined earlier.

The first issue is registration. Small-scale housing provided by a voluntary agency must be registered with the local authority to comply with the Registered Homes Act of 1984. Apart from the costs of registration, the act stipulates certain requirements which are institutionalizing in effect. For example, registered homes have to display a certificate of registration. The owner of a residential home also has to form a liaison with local fire and environmental health officers, which introduces another set of potentially institutionalizing regulations. Guidance on standards is contained in *Home life: A Code of Practice for Residential Care*.[3] In a values-based service, the aim is to provide housing which does not stand out from neighboring houses and which looks like an ordinary home. The standards imposed by the act can run counter to this aim.

However, the principle of setting external standards for the voluntary and private sectors is a good one, because it should lead to a universally higher quality of care. People leaving long-stay psychiatric hospitals have a right to good accommodations and care and need to be protected both from unscrupulous landlords and incompetent management. The important point is that appropriate standards must be developed which provide protection and enhance quality of life but do not inhibit ordinary living.

Additional constraints are imposed by planning regulations. Planning permission is not normally required for ordinary housing as some essential living areas are usually shared. It is sometimes argued that there is no change of use and that the property should be classified as a single dwelling. However, if houses are divided up into entirely self-contained units, planning permission is necessary.

Although it should be possible to have an ordinary house for two or three people classified as a single dwelling, housing providers still need to consider whether to adopt the fire and environmental health standards which are imposed on a house in multiple occupation. Some argue that these standards are institutionalizing and make the house different from other houses on the street. It is also argued that much British housing is old, of poor quality, and does not meet modern building standards. Since the aim of a residential service is to provide high-quality housing, it is better to negotiate with local officers a set of appropriate standards which are not incompatible with ordinary living.

Another dilemma is the question of whether the residents should be tenants or licensees. Tenants and licensees have different rights and status but, in general terms, tenants have the greater rights. Tenancy confers security of tenure as well as certain obligations and responsibilities. It would, therefore, seem preferable for people living in ordinary housing to become tenants. However, some housing schemes have opted for licensing because this entitles residents to claim the higher rate of board and lodging allowance from the Department of Health and Social Security (DHSS) and to slightly increase their disposable personal income. Although being classified as a licensee may bring a greater financial award, it may be socially more acceptable simply to be classified as a tenant. Whatever the interrelationship of legal requirements and planned accommodations, an effective balance must be found to ensure success for those involved.

Notes

1. A. Kay and C. Legg, "Discharged to the Community: A Review of Housing and Support for People Leaving Psychiatric Care," (London: Good Practices in Mental Health, 1986).
2. E. Bayliss, "Housing: The Foundation of Community Care," (London: MIND and National Federation of Housing Associations, 1987).
3. "Home Life: A Code of Practice for Residential Care," (London, Centre for Policy on Aging, 1984).

≈ MENTAL HEALTH AND MENTAL HEALTH SERVICES FOR BLACK AND OTHER MINORITY GROUPS

By *Parimala Moodley*

Black and other minority groups constitute about 4.5 percent of the population of the United Kingdom. Of these, the majority are in the lower socio-economic groups, have higher rates of unemployment, higher rates of homelessness, and live in run-down inner-city areas. The largest minority groups are people of West Indian origin and people of Asian origin from India, Pakistan, and Bangladesh with smaller proportions of Africans, Cypriots, Vietnamese, and Chinese.

The various groups have settled in the United Kingdom at different times and have come there for different reasons, which include those who came to work and those who came as refugees. Most minorities have tended to live together in groups, partly because they were housed together and partly because they chose to stay near each other. When these groups arrived, they suffered discrimination which continues even now. For these minority groups the data show disparate rates of mental illness, hospital admissions, and compulsory detentions.

For instance, the major features of black and other minority hospital admissions are as follows: overrepresentation in mental hospital admissions; overdiagnosis of schizophrenia; disproportionate involvement of police in admissions; higher rates of compulsory admissions and detentions; excess management in locked wards; disproportionate use of neuroleptics, or tranquilizers; and reduced follow-up with after-care services.

The studies reported by McGovern and Cope[1] in 1987 and Harrison[2] in 1988 included, for the first time, a generation of Afro-Caribbeans born or brought up from a very early age in the United Kingdom. Both studies showed high rates of schizophrenia, with the Harrison study showing a rate 12 to 14 times that of the native population. Before 1987, differences in rates were attributed to elevated hospital admission rates and variable diagnostic practices, including misdiagnoses. It was assumed that rates of mental illness would revert to some norm in successive generations just as they had for first generation immigrants. Since the 1987 and 1988 studies, there has been some radical rethinking. First, the rates have increased in the second generation, not decreased. Second, the Harrison study is an epidemiological study, not a hospital-based survey. Therefore, misdiagnosis seems to be a somewhat unlikely possibility. Even if there were substantial misdiagnoses, it should not account for rates more than ten times the rates in the native population. It would seem that there is some sort of real event, not a misdiagnosis or a miscalculation, that caused this phenomenon. Psychiatric opinion as to the nature of this event is divided between biological etiologies, such as genetic vulnerability and viral causation, and the environmental etiologies, the most alarming of which is racism.

Service provision is inextricably linked to rates of mental illness and its presentation, so service providers have to be forced to look at the disparate rates and the possible causes. There are many discrepancies between native and non-native groups which are of concern to the service providers. While many now acknowledge that services are not equitable, few are able to take up the challenge or to change the rigid methods of operating. There are, however, some examples of good practice operating within the health services.

Lynfield Mount Hospital in Bradford serves a population of 200,000; about 20 percent are immigrants or first generation descendants of immigrants from Pakistan, Bangladesh, India, Poland, and the West Indies. The transcultural psychiatry unit at Lynfield Mount Hospital is a multidisciplinary staff team which has developed expertise in transcultural issues. The staff have reasonable fluency in thirteen different languages, thereby reducing very significantly the need to use interpreters. The team works on the principle that the professionals can only be effective if they are thoroughly acquainted with the patient's background, as well as the particular stresses that minority groups are exposed to that may impinge upon daily functioning. Another example of a successful health service program is Nafsiyat, the intercultural therapy center situated in North London, which provides psychotherapy to patients who are often not accepted by other psychotherapy services. It has therapists from many different backgrounds and is prominent on the therapeutic agenda. Nafsiyat is funded by the National Health Service.

On the other hand, there are facilities which have arisen independently. Their intent has been to provide appropriate forms of care and support while seeking to challenge the racial inequalities in the health and social welfare field. The Harrambee Core and Cluster project is a black mental health project in Birmingham which has, as its theme, the development of residential accommodations for homeless black people. The project aims at dealing with far wider issues relating to psychological as well as physical needs. It works with other local groups, as well as with statutory services, to provide models of care while preserving its autonomy.

The Afro-Caribbean Mental Health Association based in South London started as a pressure group campaigning on issues of race and mental health. It now provides clinical advocacy, psychotherapy, counseling, legal advocacy, and befriending. Also in South London is the Fanon Center, a day center for blacks, that provides facilities for playing pool and listening to music, as well as for counseling, group work, adult education classes, and a West Indian-style lunch. All of these facilities provide valuable services to a neglected population. Nevertheless, hospitals continue to admit minority patients and keep them locked up.

These exemplary services seem to be providing culturally consonant, racially sensitive communication. The issue is not of separatism or integration, but of adequate and appropriate communication in its broadest sense. The way forward for all service providers is to work out what is culturally consonant and racially sensitive for the particular population served. Then the whole structure of the service will fall into place, providing balance and equity.

Providing services for black and minority patients with long-term mental health problems is particularly difficult. This is due, in part, to the nature of their problems but also in considerable part to their experience with psychiatric services that have lost credibility. The providers of psychiatric care have to meet the community on their terms. Providers have to work with the community in order to deliver the services. Unless all of those involved with mental health services can work together in a coherent fashion, there is no possibility of providing much-needed services.

Notes

1. D. McGovern and R. Cope, "First Psychiatric Admission Rates of First and Second Generation Afro-Caribbeans," *Social Psychiatry* 22 (1987), 139–49.
2. G. Harrison, D. Owen, A. Holton, D. Neilson, and D. Hoot, "A Prospective Study of Severe Mental Disorder in Afro-Caribbean Patients," *Psychological Medicine* 18, No. 3 (1988), 643–57.

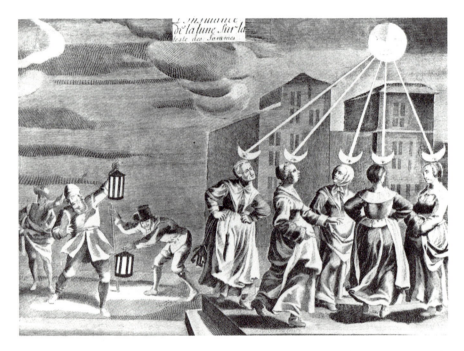

Moonstruck. From a French 17th Century Engraving; Bibl. Nat. Cab des Estamps; Courtesy of The Bettmann Archive.

∼ TRAINING FOR A NEW SERVICE

By Su Kingsley and Helen Smith

The implementation of community care will require innovative and radical shifts from established ways of working. Mental health workers will be called upon to deliver a service in very different circumstances to that of the psychiatric hospital. Training is essential if staff are to meet this challenge in a competent and creative way. Not only will the nature of the work change; relationships with other disciplines and other agencies will be different, too. One of the most striking changes will be in the relationship between staff and the people receiving services. The transition to community-based mental health services requires new and different skills and the forging of new partnerships to meet the exciting changes that lie ahead [1]

Training Goals

To be effective, a training strategy will need to reflect the values and aims of the service and a sense of how it will develop over time. Equally important, the desired characteristics of a new service should be reflected in the training that staff receive. If the new service aims to be comprehensive, coherently planned at all levels, and responsive to the changing needs of people who use it, then a training strategy should also be comprehensive, coherent, and responsive.

We have found the following fundamental principles and values helpful when thinking of service aims and objectives; they are derived from the work on normalization by Wolfensberger, O'Brien, and others: [2]

Fundamental Principles

People with disabilities:

• Have the same human value as every everyone else regardless of their degree of disability

Service Principles and Objectives

Services should:

• Provide appropriate support to person regardless of their degree of disability or dependence

- Have the same right and need to live like others in the community

- Have the same varied human needs—physical, social, and emotional—as everyone else

- Have a need and a right to a lifestyle which other citizens would value

- Be provided for in a way that does not exploit family or friends

- Support, not supplant, social networks of people with disabilities

- Be local

- Be flexible

- Be provided in the least restrictive setting possible for each person

Issues In Developing New Services

An important task facing planners and managers is to create with staff and service users a shared sense of what a community service will look like. There needs to be agreement on the values and principles underlying the service and on the aims and objectives of the service. It may seem prescriptive to state specific principles and aims, but it emphasizes the desirability of services making their goals explicit, as well as reaching a consensus with all concerned. In practice, the principles outlined above might create a service which aims to:

- Actively promote community integration by ensuring that people live and spend their time in ordinary settings;
- Maintain people's existing abilities and enhance their capacities through a coordinated program of skill learning and other activities; and
- Provide relief and stablization during times of crisis, including respite care, if necessary.

These aims could be achieved by providing people with a range of housing options using ordinary housing dispersed within a natural community. Support could be provided by a flexible staff team working with people from the base of their own homes. Rather than using segregated services (such as day hospitals/centers, lunch clubs, etc.), workers would look to ordinary community resources (such as adult education classes, leisure centers, and employment services) to help people learn new skills and build new lives.[3] Service providers might nominate a resource manager for each individual user who would ensure that a coordinated, individualized package of care is delivered when and where it should be.

Individuals who use or work in the service together with the wider community need to know about and be involved in developing these plans. This meaningful involvement in planning the service will help carry people through the difficult process of change and help create a climate of acceptance for the change.[4] Collaboration among voluntary organizations, user groups, and the local government and health authorities is crucial in building a shared vision—a vision which is paramount in providing a "marker for our destination" along what is often an uncharted and obscure path.[5]

The process of simultaneously reducing one service and building up another will be challenging for all involved. Service providers will have to work with the tension between long-term service aims and short-term goals; that is, they will have to balance what is desirable in the long term with what is necessary in the present. Everyone needs to ensure that the information needed to develop and implement the plans passes undistorted through the system. A clear picture of progress must also be communicated. Management needs to receive feedback from all levels, but especially from the point where individuals use the service in order to respond appropriately to changing needs and circumstances.[6] Therefore, plans must be flexible, not written in tablets of stone.

Involving Users In Change

For the new service providers to offer what is needed and wanted by those who will use them, the views of service users should be sought and acted upon at every stage. This involvement of people who use services has been explored in some places, especially in relation to planning. Apart from a few notable exceptions (e.g. Survivors Speak Out; Nottingham Patients Council Support Group; Glasgow LINK), user groups or individual users have rarely been involved in staff training. To effectively participate as trainers, users will need training and support—something which has often been viewed as a luxury by hard-pressed trainers. If staff are to reassess their relationship with users and focus on delivering what they really need, then users must be involved if training is to make any sense at all. There is very little literature on how best to approach this issue, but the work done on user involvement in planning may be relevant.[7]

Meeting The Needs Of Minority Ethnic Groups

A particular focus in training should be the delivery of a culturally sensitive service. Staff will need to learn what factors influence mental health work in ethnic communities. For example, the effects of racism on individuals; the higher level of social deprivation experienced by many ethnic groups; the possible conflict between dominant white values and the particular cultural and religious values of a minority ethnic community; the stress of migration; and the effects of stricter immigration laws (leading to separated families and reduced chances of marriage within the social sub-group) all have an influence on mental health work.

In particular, mental health workers need to be aware of how language is embedded in a culture and how this might lead to language being misused and misunderstood by both workers and users. The structures of our society are in many ways essentially racist, even though this is often unintentional. Workers need to explore how this can limit their professional competence. Training needs to deal with defensive maneuvers such as being overcaring; saying all people are the same and ignoring differences of race, gender and class; being over-polite; or passing individuals on to workers or voluntary organizations of the same race as a matter of course, rather than appropriateness.

Working Partnerships

New patterns of service delivery will mean new partnerships in the planning, financing, and managing of community care projects. Collaboration will help to ensure the most effective deployment of all available resources to provide a range of services matching the varied needs of users. The recent draft circular, "Collaboration between the NHS, Local Government and Voluntary Organizations," focuses on the importance of this issue, emphasizing the role of service users and caregivers and recommending their membership on joint care planning teams.[8] The total resource approach to planning advocated in this circular implies that services should be seen in their totality; a comprehensive assessment of an individual's needs would include, for example, housing and educational needs, as well as health and personal social services.

The implication of these recommendations is that staff at all levels will need to familiarize themselves with the ways other organizations work. They will also need to be encouraged to make links with groups they have not traditionally worked with, such as adult education and housing departments. For minority ethnic groups, it might also be important to work with the institutions which maintain the culture and religion of the community, such as temples and mosques.

Working across traditional organizational boundaries will also require more flexible financial arrangements. This, in itself, presents a challenge to planners, managers, and finance staff who will need to find creative ways of working together to provide resources for new schemes. Other sources of finance to joint funding need to be exploited, including urban program money, housing associations (for capital finance), voluntary sector grant funding, and social security payments. There are already some instances where the management of finance is adapting to more complex situations as, for example, in the development of consortia.[9]

Effective community care implies teamwork or a multi-disciplinary/multi-agency approach. The needs of people using the mental health service are so varied that no one person, profession, or agency can provide all the necessary help and support. Drawing on a wide range of professional and personal abilities increases the chances for an individual to receive appropriate help and support.

The problem with most existing professional training is that focusing on a particular profession can create impermeable boundaries around each discipline, perpetuating the idea that each discipline has knowledge and skills inaccessible to other disciplines. This is not a good basis for developing new services which require inter-professional working and collaboration. Such boundaries may lead to increased opportunities for conflict and rivalry, and may provoke difficulties in working with non-professionals, such as users and volunteers. At worst, they can limit the options available to individuals and restrict their access to other types of help and support.

Working in a team is a skill that needs to be learned and developed. Staff who have traditionally felt their primary loyalties were to their profession may find it difficult to work effectively in a multi-disciplinary team. Professionals who have tended to be in control, such as psychiatrists, may also find it difficult to share their power.

Teamwork will probably be encouraged best by the development of joint training with a focus on shared issues. The audit commission's report on community care noted the importance of new working practices and recommended that "the concept of a core of community health skills could be developed for all those involved in community-based care, based on shared training."[10] The report proposed initial training for basic grade care workers who would provide general support and act as the main contact for people in the community. This first level of training could then be supplemented with the acquisition of specific skills, enabling workers to become more specialized in particular aspects of community care or in the needs of specific client groups. These proposals would complement multi-disciplinary work by encouraging a generalist approach to mental health work, based on meeting individual needs rather than working from particular professional perspectives. This approach may also highlight personal abilities, such as good negotiating skills and keeping calm in a crisis, as equally important aspects of doing the job. Training for those who work in new community services will need to focus more on what is really needed at the point of service delivery and less on professional distinctions.

New Ways Of Looking At Training

Effective training must grow from and be founded in the principles and aims of service development. Training should help ensure that the services people use come as close as possible to the goals jointly accepted by users and providers and that these goals are open to continual challenge. In this way, services will continue to move forward. But there are also some key values and principles which need to underpin the way training takes place. Previously, most training in the caring professions has been based on the acquisition of knowledge within specific professional disciplines (e.g. nursing, social work, medicine, and psychology). For many workers, training has been concentrated at the beginning of their careers, followed by rare opportunities for time off to acquire some particular practice skill.

Many people currently working in psychiatric hospitals will need re-training opportunities to equip them with new skills to work in community settings and to assist them in successfully negotiating what will be a major life change. This means paying attention to both the skills and the emotional implications.

There is a danger that if training is based too heavily on traditional models of education, this will leave learners in a dependent relationship with the trainer/teacher. If not encouraged to take the initiative, they may not know how to transfer their knowledge to new and complex situations outside the classroom. The emotional components associated with change—anxiety, uncertainty, and fear—may also not be addressed. This could be prevented if participants themselves took more responsibility for defining what and how they learned and if training focused as much on experiential as on knowledge-based learning, such as formal lectures. An example is the training initiative associated with the housing support team which helps people make the transition from homeless to householder status.[11] The courses start by brainstorming the sorts of changes participants anticipate, and continue with building the training program around the needs that these changes will bring.[12]

In other settings, learner-centered approaches to training have been used to develop participants' ability to carry over learning to new situations and to learn from experience. Key features include the following: an orientation which stresses the present and the future, rather than concentrating on what can be analyzed from the past; objectives set by the learner; a focus on questioning rather than on knowing the correct answers; and the exploration of feelings and anxieties which may help learners take risks in new settings.[13] Rather than acquiring specific knowledge and narrow skills, this approach aims to develop people's overall skills as learned from experience.

Using this framework, it is possible to draw up a set of objectives aimed at training for transition to community services which include the following:

- Identifying the needs of all people who will use the services;
- Extending opportunities for service users to participate as equal members in developing plans and running training events;
- Enabling workers to acquire the specific skills of planning with individuals, helping people become more independent, keeping records, managing resources, dealing with the public, and so on;
- Helping staff and service users accept and be involved in service changes;
- Maintaining morale by ensuring that staff continue to feel valued;
- Communicating all relevant policy decisions;
- Enabling people to cope better with uncertainty, ambiguity, and relative answers;
- Creating a vision of the new service which provides a purpose and a framework for identifying new skills, such as knowledge of welfare benefits and housing regulations, along with counseling skills, working with people in crisis, and so on;

- Helping people to identify and use their own skills and existing resources;
- Identifying and turning to advantage the constraints to change;
- Restructuring and learning from past experience, especially the effects on the lives of users and workers of past services, in order to overcome prejudices;
- Providing an opportunity for people to explore attitudes, values, and feelings while increasing their awareness of the effects of these on their own and others' behavior;
- Clarifying roles within the new services with an emphasis on teambuilding and enhancing cooperative problem solving; and
- Creating a plan of action that is connected with the wider service developments.[14]

In designing effective new services, similar opportunities need to be made available to staff. Training is an important vehicle for opening up such opportunities. However, training will only be helpful if individuals feel that their effectiveness is improved. When this happens, training is empowering. However, staff need opportunities to explore feelings, attitudes, and personal values, as well as skills and knowledge, for this empowerment to occur.

Different Dimensions Of Learning

Personal change in working practice is dependent upon an individual's knowledge, understanding, beliefs, and attitudes. Training needs to take account of all these, providing a balance of activities which allows people to develop an increasingly greater sense of their own competence. The possibility of feeling one's skills are inadequate for working in the community leads to lack of confidence, low self-esteem, and the erection of barriers to further learning and development. Hospital rundown or closure and the need to move into the community means that many staff currently working in mental health services are facing this fear. Acquiring competence in new skills enhances self-esteem and motivates people to gain further competence.

The proposed model of staff training and development is based on four key elements: knowledge, understanding, values, and attitudes. Figure 1 illustrates this model. The model is circular to emphasize the interaction among the different elements. Each term has a specific meaning. This is an interactive model even though key elements have been defined separately for ease of explanation.

A Model For Personal Change

Knowledge includes the acquisition and mastery of information. It may be obtained by generalizing from experience, but it is usually learned formally from books, lectures, or observation. Knowledge is often transmitted in concepts which

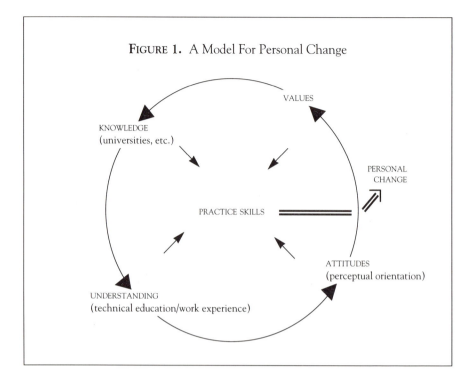

FIGURE 1. A Model For Personal Change

VALUES

KNOWLEDGE
(universities, etc.)

PERSONAL
CHANGE

PRACTICE SKILLS

ATTITUDES
(perceptual orientation)

UNDERSTANDING
(technical education/work experience)

link up with theories about the world and, as such, is not value-free. For example, hypotheses about the cause of schizophrenia differ. The medical model is based on an individual's having no control over an invasive or inherited disease, while the dynamic, interpersonal model is based on the belief that early childhood experiences are of primary importance.

Treatment of schizophrenia depends upon what is accepted as knowledge about the cause. In the examples above, treatment would range from phenothiazine medication to psychoanalysis or family therapy. The choice of a medical or interpersonal conceptualization of schizophrenia can be influenced by other more general theories an individual might hold. For example, someone who believes in fate and predestination is more likely to view schizophrenia as a disease over which there is no control. On the other hand, someone who functions as an active agent in the world might believe that the resolution of mental distress is within his or her own power. This is a crude distinction, but serves to show how knowledge is expressed in concepts which are linked with many other individual beliefs.

Theories about knowledge itself are rare; however, Terry[15] suggests that there are nine levels. The first few levels are defined as absolutism where people believe there is a right and a wrong solution to a problem. The mid-range is relativism, where people believe that all approaches have equal viability or validity. The final range and the most sophisticated is relativism with commitment in which an individual believes there are different ways of looking at a problem but chooses an approach which suits him/her best.

In training staff, it is important to uncover their levels of knowledge in order to help them understand the nature of the training. If staff are waiting to be told the "right answer," which is Terry's absolutism, then they are unlikely to benefit much from training or service where there are few right answers.

Understanding is the application of knowledge or an ability to act appropriately on the basis of knowledge. For instance, using knowledge to solve problems or contribute to discussions both involve understanding. Understanding is the difference between just repeating knowledge and using it to extend the range of things one can do with it. For example, a worker may know what questions to ask when assessing an individual. Yet the ability to choose appropriately from a range of treatment/action options depends upon an understanding of why these particular questions are asked and the implication of the answers. Understanding often develops through the experience of putting the knowledge into practice.

Values or basic beliefs are personal moral codes which indicate what we accept as right and wrong, and consequently determine how we act in different situations. Basic beliefs may make us more receptive to some aspects of knowledge and more resistant to others. For example, if we believe that long-term hospital residents retain basic citizenship rights, we are more likely to support efforts to rehouse people in the community than if we believe that they have lost their ability to be contributing members of society.

Some readers may be concerned about our inclusion of basic beliefs in this model. Training methods have been used in the last 20 years which appear to rely heavily on breaking down defenses and shattering basic beliefs. One example is Erhard Seminar Training (EST). Some compare these methods to brainwashing techniques. These techniques are not being advocated, but it is important to examine and identify the basic beliefs of the trainer and the learner, since these will influence receptivity to new knowledge. Research has shown that the results of children's I.Q. tests are influenced by what the teacher administering the tests has been told about individual children, especially in regard to their social class. In other words, our assumptions and beliefs can limit the success of others—a pertinent lesson for mental health workers who may be unwittingly restricting the lives of service users through their beliefs about users' abilities.

Those concerned with addressing basic beliefs should examine the assumptions and attitudes inherent in existing professional training. This is important if trainers are to be clear about the beliefs underpinning their new training; otherwise, those involved in retraining may remain unaware of the basic beliefs originally learned when they became mental health workers.

In developing new patterns of services for people traditionally seen as patients or passive recipients of care, it is crucial that staff in those services spend time examining their beliefs about service users, and their assumptions about users' needs, capacities, attributes, and rights. Workers also need to explore their beliefs about people from different races and cultural backgrounds. This exploration may reveal lack of knowledge about different lifestyles, and lack of understanding of certain aspects of a culture, such as the significance of religious rituals. Basic beliefs about people who use services will influence how staff make sense of the move to the community and how they respond to any training program.

Attitudes involve emotions and affect the way we feel about new ideas in relation to our values. For instance, experiencing success in previously difficult activities brings confidence and pleasure to exercising newfound skills. Dealing with deep-seated prejudices can also improve our working and personal relationships with other people. For example, discovering that an individual, institutionalized for many years, has retained a love of music may give him/her something in common with a member of the staff. The staff member can communicate with the person through music and be pleased if successful. This experience may encourage the worker to seek different ways of communicating with other individuals in the ward and may change the worker's perception of the users as severely damaged people with nothing to contribute to others.

Practice skills are the vehicle for action. The practice of new skills is a demonstration of competence through knowledge and understanding and may also indicate changes in basic beliefs and attitudes. For example, someone successfully facilitating a self-advocacy group may demonstrate knowledge of the concepts of self-advocacy and an understanding of the sensitive role of staff in this process. This role may also indicate a shift in basic beliefs, for instance, that users have the right to exercise self-advocacy. Any subsequent success of the group will serve to further develop the staff's practical skills in supporting and encouraging users to take up self-advocacy. Finally this may further encourage a change in attitudes, such as the idea that this is a good and positive thing to pursue.

For training to be effective, interventions must be planned which address each and every aspect appropriately. Simply teaching people new skills will not be useful if they do not also have knowledge about appropriate use of the technique and the basic belief that this is a relevant practice. On the other hand, giving people knowledge without the means to use it in practice makes learning an academic exercise which quickly loses all relevance to the real world.

Principles Into Practice

Examples of good training models are given later which seek to incorporate many of the factors discussed above. First, it will be useful to examine an established training exercise and look at how it fits the model. Program Analysis of Service Systems (PASS) is a training exercise devised to enable people to evaluate services for people with disabilities.[16] It was originally developed for use in service to people with learning difficulties, but is now also being used by people working in mental health as well as in other services concerned with disabilities. PASS is a good way to enable people to understand the impact of services on their lives and provide a practical framework for service design. It is a complex tool which demands awareness and sensitivity from those who use it. In order to maintain its high standards, PASS training materials are not available off the shelf. PASS is taught through residential workshops, typically stretching over an intensive five- to six-day period.

The workshops are designed to familiarize participants with the widely accepted theory of normalization and its practical implications as first developed in the United States in the 1970s by Wolfensberger, O'Brien, and others.[17] By the end of the workshop, participants should understand how it can be used and applied in practice, and they should have had practical experience in doing this. They will have been challenged to examine their own underlying beliefs and value systems in the light of normalization and will have had an opportunity to reconsider their attitudes at the points where they experience significant conflict. Different aspects are addressed during a PASS training workshop.

Personal Changes: Working with PASS can lead to personal change through confronting and challenging beliefs and attitudes. As the workshop progresses, participants are required to interact with service users in a way which almost certainly differs from their normal working role. For a much longer period than is usual in professional contacts, they spend time getting to know users. There is no structured brief and participants are encouraged to get to know users as people with likes and dislikes, a past history, aspirations, and future plans. In this way, the workshop often challenges the legitimacy of the knowledge and understanding gained through professional training. Previously held assumptions about users' capabilities, life experiences, and potential to contribute to society are in question after meeting people outside the usual staff-patient/client relationship.

Basic Beliefs: Participants in a PASS workshop are introduced at an early stage to the clearly stated beliefs and principles that form the value base for the workshop. Normalization is based on the premise that each individual is of equal human value, regardless of disability. This basic belief generates other fundamental principles and service principles based on human rights and dignity. The rest of the workshop flows from these principles, and participants are constantly reminded of their importance and asked to consider the implications for working practice.

Knowledge: The theory of normalization which is the basis of PASS is concerned with notions of what is typically valued by people in our society. Examples include a house, job, good health, and wealth. It shows how people with disabilities become devalued by losing these assets through their experience. Sociological theories, in particular deviancy theory, are used to demonstrate how the good intentions of many human service workers are constrained by attitudes and practices which are widespread throughout society. The workshop looks at how services themselves can become handicaps for people with disabilities. Contact with the service may restrict an individual's access to a valued lifestyle by actually controlling that lifestyle. This may occur through confinement to a long-term hospital or through the secondary stigma associated with service contact, such as difficulties in finding a job because of having a psychiatric record.

Knowledge is presented in the workshop through written material to be read prior to attending the workshop and lecture sessions involving all participants with extensive use of audio-visual aids. The workshop is structured so that these education sessions are interspersed over the five days, building on and contributing to an increasing level of understanding.

Understanding: PASS workshops aim at developing an understanding of how services affect people's lives. Understanding is aided by the use of newly acquired knowledge to undertake a practice evaluation of a simulated service. The effects of reaching agreement on the rating of one aspect of the service helps participants develop an understanding of how the beliefs, values, and theories may be put into practice. A major part of the workshop is a visit to a real service site where participants get to know the people using that service. This exercise serves to increase understanding about the impact of the service on people's lives and helps participants focus more strongly on users.

Attitudes: Personal views may be reinforced or changed by PASS. The training challenges workers' attitudes, not just towards the particular group of people they normally work with, but towards all disadvantaged groups. The small teams in which participants work provide a safe, intimate environment for them to explore their views about people who receive services. Attitudes are challenged in this setting through increased discussion and debate with other participants and the group facilitator.

Practice Skills: PASS workshops do not directly address working practices. The aim of the workshops is to help people examine their beliefs and values, rather than teach them new skills. However, participants may well review the relevance of their existing work skills. In this way, PASS helps individuals identify what sorts of skills they need to learn in order to work in a community service.

A Strategy For Training

If community psychiatric services are to provide significantly improved opportunities in the lives of service users, staff will require considerable training input. Training programs will have to address a range of different needs in terms of both professional background and seniority in the organization. Programs will also need to support inter-agency coordination, working much more explicitly than professional training is currently able to do. Training will need to be carried out at regular intervals throughout a worker's career. Training should provide continuing developmental support and play an important role in the continuing evolution of the service. The multi-dimensional and long-term nature of such training suggests that a strategic approach will be required for effectiveness.

Defining Strategy

Strategy is a word that takes on many different meanings. The definition of strategy which we have found helpful is "an activity which combines a number of areas of work in a way which multiplies their individual effectiveness and gives clear direction." This activity needs to be based on clearly stated values which are reflected in the goals of the organization. For example, a successful strategy to resettle people from a psychiatric hospital into the community must coordinate a range of voluntary, statutory, and ordinary community services, including housing, support in crisis, leisure, and welfare benefits which offer a comprehensive service to individual users. It will only be successful if there is a clear, agreed-upon definition of what constitutes a good service and what is a desirable outcome. In this way, a strategy helps organizations, groups, or individuals to achieve and improve their outcomes.[18]

By this definition, strategy must be explicitly related to the organization's goals and values, usually expressed through various policy statements. Thus, organizational policy should provide the foundation for a training strategy, and the strategy for training should represent the organization's plans for making its policies effective. The bestseller, *In Search of Excellence*, by Waterman and Peters, discusses the question of strategy in relation to successful private companies whose strategies and structures were driven by changing pressures in the market place.[19] The equivalent driving force in health service training should ideally be the organizational policy which reflects the needs and requirements of people who use services. In an actual training practice, strategy may sometimes be based on organizational needs only, turning it into an instrument of management so that training improves the way the organization runs but not the service offered.[20]

In an ideal training strategy there are likely to be at least two main streams of activity: the first directed towards communicating the organization's goals, policies, and values with encouragement of a wider ownership and understanding; and the second focused on developing the practical capacities of staff in the organization to achieve those goals. Management must ensure that training takes place, and that it is valued and supported. It is important to emphasize this last point because too often training appears to be a substitute for managerial action which is expected to resolve problems within the organization.[21] On the contrary, for training to be effective, management must keep pace with the organizational changes which training programs are addressing. There is no point in training staff to work in community settings if the other aspects of building up a community service are not also being pursued.

A Strategy Checklist

Key questions which need to be answered when devising a training strategy include the following:

- What is the purpose of training?
- How can training assist the fulfillment of the organization's objectives?
- What kinds of training already exist?

- Who is responsible for training?
- What is the intended scope of the training program? Will it include different agencies, professions, grades, service delivery settings, or individual needs?
- How can a favorable context for training be created, especially in relation to service development plans?

This last point is particularly important. Training has often concentrated on improving individual skills with little reference to how or when these new skills can be practiced.[22]

Taking cognizance of these points, the training strategy for the Wells Road service for people with learning difficulties focused on six conditions for creating a healthy context for training:

- The integration of training activities into the planning process and day-to-day management activities;
- The investment of real resources such as a commitment to provide space and time for learning;
- The identification of where staff are starting from through individualized program plans;
- Defining the key role of line managers plus equipping them with appropriate skills as trainers within their own staff groups;
- Ensuring that the appropriate personnel and management support activities are in place; and
- Ensuring appropriate time frameworks for the program, as they relate to different groups of staff.[23]

A Value Base For Training

Our model of adult learning suggests that we need to pay equal attention to identifying value systems and attitudes, as well as inculcating knowledge and developing competence. The values which inform service plans and contribute to the goals of a service should be applied to every aspect of training. Therefore, if service development is to be based on the principle of normalization, an important value and goal for the service will be respect for each user as an individual. In the same way, those training staff members must also treat them with respect and value their individuality. If this does not happen, then it is extremely unlikely that an undervalued staff will be able to provide the respect and attention that the service is trying to achieve for its users.

There are five key aspects to a training strategy for transition. The first is taking multiple interests into account. The development of community-based mental health services depends upon the involvement of a wide range of service-providing agencies in the voluntary sector, as well as upon health and local authorities. It will also require the services of staff from a broad range of professional backgrounds and experience. A training strategy will first need to identify all voluntary and statutory agencies likely to be contributing to the service. Second, it will need to define the range of professionally trained people whose skills and expertise will be relevant to training resources. For example, hospital-based staff will need help in developing community work skills. Field staff may need help in working with people in local residential settings. Staff from these areas of work could assist in training others from different settings. Third, a training strategy should identify the different needs of different grades of staff. Unskilled and junior staff will need training to move into the community. Senior professional staff and managers will need training in new ways to support and manage their staff. The fourth need is to describe the support required to cope with the changes. The early stages of change may be easier for care staff if they are involved in planning the new services. The more complex forms of joint management and control of services which may evolve later will require managers to develop new ways of working with other staff and other agencies. Being involved in the planning process may help alleviate anxiety.

The second key aspect to a training strategy is in meeting multiple individual needs with a limited range of available resources. One solution would be to design an appropriate package for individual users, utilizing the range of resources available through individual planning to meet staff training needs.[24] An individual plan will need to include an assessment of the individual's current strengths and areas in which one hopes to develop new skills to improve performance. The plan would be worked out with the individual and would identify how help could be provided through training, either within the organization or using external resources. Finally, the plan would be designed to achieve some specific objectives over a specified time period. Both the individual staff member and their line managers would need to agree to the plan at the beginning of a regular appraisal process.

In this way, staff could be provided with opportunities to identify their developmental interests and the areas in which their competence needs to be enhanced if they are to participate fully in the new service. These individual training needs could then be met through a modular training program. This might include some elements for all staff, some elements for selected or project-based staff, and some individual elements met through participation in further education or the use of distance-learning materials such as open university packages/courses.

A third key factor is using multiple locations. Training should not take place through a single course provided in a uniform way. The great majority of training officers who replied to our survey stated that their major training resource was in-house programs, but there was generally little use of other local and national resources. We envision that a training strategy would consider using local and regional resources available through colleges, universities, and other training agencies. It would also include considerable elements of internal training. Some of this would be in the form of yard courses run by outsiders. Some would be seminars and specific skill-related courses provided locally. Some would relate to staff teams or individuals working alongside other teams in their work settings to provide actual on-the-job training.

In addition to these activities, we would expect people periodically to be sent to national workshops and seminars and to be supported in their access to individual learning packages, whether through the open university, open technical school, national extension college, or other bodies. Finally, local resources of literature, self-instructional material, and videos would provide a valuable support to individual learning.

Ensuring continuity and responsibility is a fourth key factor in training strategy. Training needs to be related equally to the developmental needs of staff and the services they are working in, but neither of these areas is static. Consequently, training must be sustained over time, continuously identifying and meeting new needs which arise in response to new ideas and demands. In this way, training can help the service remain alive and vivid rather than becoming ossified and stale. Maintaining and improving the quality of the service is closely related to training. Thus, part of a quality assurance strategy for new services should be the creation of a system of in-service training which links continued service development with continuous staff development. Training is as much a responsibility of the service managers as it is of the training department, and the two must work together to address the organization's needs.

Finally, the resources for training are of key importance. Training as a major element in service development will inevitably require adequate resources, and any strategy must include careful consideration of these implications. Clearly, training has direct financial costs, whether internal, external, or individual learning is involved.

Trainers need to be planners and managers of training programs, as well as providers of direct training.[25] The training program will also need to indicate where training is to be delivered and whether initial training will then enable the recipients to train other staff. A variety of local, regional, and national training providers will need to be identified.

In order to make the best use of these various opportunities, training packages to meet individual staff needs will have to be carefully designed and supported through sensitive staff appraisal. For staff to benefit fully from off-the-job training, adequate coverage arrangements will be necessary to release them from their day-to-day responsibilities.

A Training Checklist

The framework of an active training plan should consider the following questions:
- Will there be a conscious process of identifying the demands which new patterns of service delivery will place on staff?
- Will training reflect the same values and goals as those which underpin the service development strategy?
- Will ways of involving service users in training programs be identified and utilized?

- Will the training strategy address the need to create a cultural shift within the organization in order to reflect new values and goals?
- Will appropriate training programs be planned for all grades of staff throughout the organization?
- Will training specifically address how staff can deliver a culturally and ethnically sensitive service?
- Will training be geared to identifying and meeting individual staff needs through individual programs built up from a range of resources?
- Will training plans provide for a continuing process of staff development and service evaluation?
- Will training be shared with other relevant agencies such as:
  health authorities;
  local authority social services;
  housing associations;
  voluntary groups such as MIND, National Schizophrenia Fellowship, Richmond Fellowship, Mental After-Care Association (and many more local groups);
  adult education services; and
  voluntary black and ethnic minority groups and community leaders?
- Will training be an integral part of a strategy for managing change within the mental health service?
- Will the resource requirements for training be identified, and will there be ways of meeting these needs?
- Will the training strategy utilize a range of resources and locations both inside and outside the organization?

Proposal For A Model District Training Strategy

Addressing the issues we have outlined above will demand a comprehensive initiative, involving a broad range of interests and being innovative and experimental in the type of training made available. Such an initiative needs to be developed with the participation of a wide range of people who are involved in and affected by the changes in services. The initiative should also be able to experiment with new approaches and to learn from these. There are many ways to develop training strategies which meet these criteria. However, a new model has been created which suggests one way of planning a district strategy. The model has several stages and starts with an assessment of new service requirements and existing staff potential.

It is important to recognize that neither training needs, staff's abilities, or their expectations of what the service will provide are static pieces of information. Rather they are likely to be in flux and will require rechecking regularly in order to ensure that training is on course and is reoriented to changing needs.

Having made some preliminary assessment of training requirements, the train-

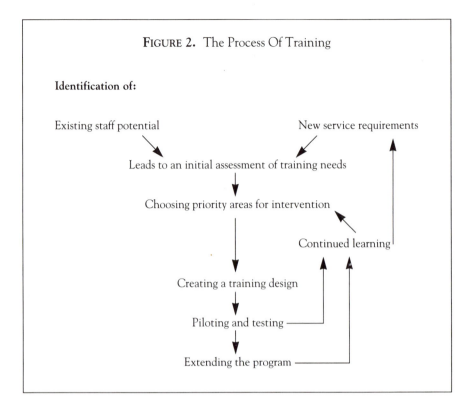

FIGURE 2. The Process Of Training

Identification of:

Existing staff potential   New service requirements

Leads to an initial assessment of training needs

Choosing priority areas for intervention

Continued learning

Creating a training design

Piloting and testing

Extending the program

ing strategy will need to determine where interventions are going to be targeted for maximum impact. Training needs should be prioritized to ensure that the most urgent requirements are addressed first, allowing staff to tackle other areas in order of significance. Piloting and testing are a further necessary stage in the process. This enables the design to be tested before extending it district-wide. Modifications and alterations should be made at this stage, possibly leading to a reassessment of service requirements or another look at the training design. The stages of this model are represented in Figure 2, which shows diagramatically the process of devising a training strategy. At the same time, staff will be going through these experimental training programs and should already be deriving benefit from them.

The Process Of Training

The overall program will then continue to develop along these lines, being extended to different groups of staff and to new projects. The program should be constantly responsive to feedback from participants, both during training and as they become better able to assess the relevance of training in their new work roles and workplaces.

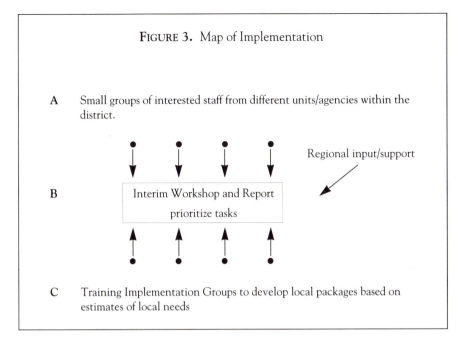

FIGURE 3. Map of Implementation

A   Small groups of interested staff from different units/agencies within the district.

Regional input/support

B   Interim Workshop and Report prioritize tasks

C   Training Implementation Groups to develop local packages based on estimates of local needs

Implementing The Training Program

It is inappropriate for a single individual or agency to take on the whole task of devising a training strategy. The strategy should be developed and implemented by multi-disciplinary and multi-agency groups, working together within a coordinated framework and developing a shared ownership of the strategy. This will inevitably require energetic and sophisticated leadership, but we do not think it is important which agency provides such leadership. What matters is that whoever leads the process has the capacity to communicate a vision of the future and is able to generate commitment to joint working and joint problem-solving from the different parties involved. The map in Figure 3 illustrates the implementation stages of the program.

Stage One—Training Assessment Groups

The first stage (A on Figure 3) is to establish small groups to identify training needs. These groups are likely to include interested staff from all the appropriate units/workplaces in both health and social service agencies within a district, as well as professional and lay members of local voluntary organizations. There is also a strong case for including users, unpaid caregivers, and a variety of other members of the community in these groups. Their tasks would include determining the skills needed in the new service, assessing the existing staff potential, and identifying alternative sources of staff.

The groups have three key tasks in this initial phase. First, the abilities and potential of the present staff group should be assessed including their skills, interests, and preferences. The groups should also be finding out how workers perceive their own developmental needs and linking them to the district plans for the new service. Second, an assessment should be made of what the new service will require in the way of training. Using service development plans to identify the new skills that will be needed during the transition to community-based services will be a key function of the multi-disciplinary groups in this first phase. Third, alternative and additional sources of skills should be explored. Individuals bring with them particular skills which will be useful in the new service.

In some districts it may be simplest to set up three task forces, each taking on one of the above functions. In other districts it may be better to have four or five groups, each handling all the functions but covering a specific geographical area. There are likely to be a number of different ways of arranging this, and we do not think that at this stage one method can be identified as the best. The most important thing is to ensure that whatever way is chosen best fits the local situation both structurally and politically.

In summary, during the initial phase, multi-disciplinary and multi-agency groups will be required to:

- Identify the underlying philosophy and tasks of the new service to be provided;
- Define the skills and staff required to make this service a viable proposition; and
- Explore available options for finding and training staff, including remotivating existing staff and identifying potential new pools of personnel.

Setting up these groups may have to be done initially by one or two enthusiasts who can motivate others to join in drawing up a district-wide strategy.

Stage Two—Workshop And Interim Report

As the groups make progress on these tasks, the next stage (B on Figure 3) will consist of a joint workshop for all local stakeholders in present and future services. The workshop will provide an opportunity to broaden participation and to strengthen local involvement. It will provide an early opportunity for those unable to commit time to the initial working groups to contribute to the design and development of the training strategy. The participants at the workshop should include representatives from voluntary organizations, ethnic communities, and user groups. The workshop must be comprehensive both in content and range of people attending; otherwise the priorities that emerge may be skewed and unhelpful.

The workshop would aim to do the following:

- Provide feedback to each of the small groups on the appropriateness and usefulness of their proposals, especially in the light of work done by the other groups;
- Negotiate overall training aims and objectives for the district to pursue;
- Decide upon training priorities; and
- Prepare for further training activities by establishing the value of a strategic approach and reaching a consensus of approval and understanding of the proposed training program.

Regional support may need to be sought at this stage and the use of regional resources discussed. A report stating the findings of the small groups and the agreed priorities would be useful to circulate to those unable to attend as well as to use for future reference.

Stage Three—Training Implementation Groups

Stage three proposes the creation of a new set of working groups (C on Figure 3). These groups could be based on the previous small groups, although it is not necessary to do so. If not done already, membership should be extended beyond staff to include service users, representatives of voluntary organizations, and other appropriate people in line with the priorities set by the workshop. At this stage, they are more likely to look like a task force network, and they could be regarded as training implementation groups. Their task would be to devise local ways to meet training needs based on estimates of local need as assessed by the small groups, and determine the overall direction and priorities decided in the workshop and mandated at a regional level.

Implementation training groups could take as their initial focus some new service development, such as a specific project. Their task would be to identify and assess the training needs for staff coming to work in the project, both in terms of the skills needed in order to deliver the service effectively and the developmental needs of individual staff. This latter task may not always be possible if staff are new and not coming from other parts of the service. They will need to design ways of meeting these needs and this may require a variety of interventions.

Some training will be needed which brings the whole project staff together. A session to determine philosophies and modes of working together as a community mental health team is one way to do it. Individual staff members may need to participate in district-wide training, and there may also be a case for sending some staff on to existing training programs offered by educational agencies. A community work course at a local college, or support for one of the open university community care programs are examples of relevant options. Finally, it may also be deemed necessary to improve the general professional competence of staff, through specialized nurse training or social work courses. Examples of training needs and possible service responses are shown in Figure 4.

Stage Four—Training Network

The training implementation groups could form a district network both providing mutual support and anticipating future training requirements. Regular meetings of members of the network could form an exciting and creative forum for maintaining awareness of changing training needs and stimulating new ways of meeting those needs. In this way, an element of continual development would be provided for the service as a whole, offering a forum in which problems could be aired and new ideas proposed.

Training In Action

Some training strategies which seem to be examples of good practice have been included here.

Wigan Health Authority has created a training program based on a multi-disciplinary approach. It is using line managers as trainers, which enables training to be closely related to the workplace and provides for individual development in conjunction with the staff appraisal system. There are three key principles underlying the training program:

- Focus on individual staff needs and development;
- Skills taught should clearly reflect client needs; and
- Training stimulates staff to continue developing their skills, and enables staff to pass these on to other staff.

The program spans the whole staff group and includes: initial induction training; basic occupational training; training for individual performance appraisal; development of training skills in staff; supervisor development; and management training. The content of training is clearly related to the need for new skills and increased awareness of what is required by the move to community-based services. It includes elements provided in-house together with external training.

South Lincolnshire Health Authority established a multi-disciplinary staff training group in 1985, focusing on the problems created by organizational change and the decentralization of services. The aims of the group were to help staff understand and cope with changes in both National Health Service management

FIGURE 4. Examples of Training Needs and Responses in a New Service

Staff will need to develop new:
- relationships with colleagues and service users
- attitudes and expectations
- skills
- knowledge about service users and service models

Managers will need to develop new:
- expectations of staff
- planning and implementation skills
- performance measures
- leadership skills
- development roles

Some training needs:
- knowledge and information about new services
- community/neighborhood work skills
- support for learning from experience
- team development
- ability-focused assessment
- goal setting

Some possible responses; project level:
- induction courses
- teamwork support

district level:
- values workshop
- skill development

regionwide:
- supplements to education
- programs
- management development

and in mental health provision and to provide a means of minimizing speculation and anxiety concerning the future of the mental health service.

The group has organized an initial one-day workshop, bringing together key staff in middle and first-line management from health, social services, voluntary agencies, housing, the probation service, and the police. This workshop was devised and run by external consultants, but similar events have since been organized by district staff. These local events are preceded by a questionnaire sent to participants which asks for their expectations of, and views on, prospective changes in the service. It also asks staff to speculate on the opportunities this could provide for them, together with their own assessment of their current training needs in order to make the most of these opportunities. The workshops are also being supported by training in managerial, technical, and job-related skills. In addition, the group produces a regular news sheet, giving details of training activities and resources.

Torbay Health Authority and South Devon Social Services have developed a joint strategy providing interdisciplinary education for both professionals and volunteers involved with mental health services. The first two years of this joint inservice training program included reorientation courses for staff moving from hospital to community services; development courses to improve existing standards of practice; specialization skills for experienced practitioners with an emphasis on the practical application skills; workshops on topics of general interest in mental health; and special interest groups providing an opportunity for small groups to develop while being supported in testing out new ideas. Volunteer counselors are trained to work cooperatively with or independent of the statutory services. The present focus is on providing a psychotherapy course and more specialist education.

In addition, Torbay has an innovative approach to basic RMN training, based on adult education principles where learners take a major part in determining their learning needs. The key to this is the attachment of learners to existing staff who act as mentors. This enables much greater flexibility about placements and the pace of learning, and provides a structure for individual support. The intention is to produce staff who are much better fitted for new roles in the developing community services.

Kirklees Partnership in Community Care is a collaborative group consisting of Huddersfield and Dewsbury Health Authorities, Kirklees Metropolitan Council Social Services Department, and various voluntary organizations. One element of their work is represented by the Project Working Group on Training and Staff Development, which has set up a multi-disciplinary course to facilitate the development of community-based mental health services. The course aims to enable participants to develop effective teamwork within inter-disciplinary teams. The focus is on developing helping skills based on the belief that whatever roles people play in community services (seeking or giving help, or supervising), personal relationships are the key to success. Participants are encouraged to set their own goals for learning and to evaluate whether they are being helped to achieve these as the course progresses. Themes in the course include the following:

- Exploring values and attitudes;
- Solving problems and making decisions;

- Examining conflicts of interest;
- Scanning roles;
- Examining the progress of community care; and
- Reflecting, evaluating, and planning for the future.

South East Thames Regional Health Authority in conjunction with the University of Kent has built a regional team of trainers, practitioners, and researchers who are working with health and local authorities in the region to support the transition from large institutions to local services. As well as working with individual authorities to develop local training packages, the team has created a number of special regional initiatives which address specific training needs and which are pioneering and testing new ways to support service development. These courses and workshops are open to people working in health or social services departments, education services, and voluntary agencies. They are intentionally multi-disciplinary and stress the links between training and service development through project work and supervised local training initiatives. Much of the work of the regional team is designed to train trainers, which will strengthen local competence to deal with staff development issues rather than take over that function.

This work has focused on services for people with learning difficulties, but the regional team is now expanding into mental health services. The training strategy used in both areas combines organizational development with training targeted at individuals. The main areas of work dealing with learning difficulties include the following categories:

Defining Exemplary Service Models

A special course, "Developing Staffed Housing for People with Mental Handicaps," (1983–85), was able to draw on the available knowledge and experience of staffed housing services for people with severe and profound learning difficulties. Recently, a special development team has been set up to help local services create a good quality of life for people with learning difficulties and challenging behavior by giving extra help through staff with the experience, time, knowledge, and resources to provide assistance.

Training The Trainers

A framework entitled "Joint Assessment of Local Training Need" has been set up to review local training needs across agencies and disciplines in order to produce local training strategies. A trainers' development program is run each year to equip local staff with the skills to implement local training strategies. Six modern training packages for front-line staff have been produced to meet the need for effective materials. Special workshops have also been offered on the organization of community teams, policies and guidelines dealing with sex-based behavior and biases, and using open university resources.

Individual Training And Development

A two-year part-time masters degree program has been set up at the University of Kent designed specifically for people who will lead the development of community care. In addition, two proposals have been developed for shared training of nurses and social services staff. One of these has now received approval from the validating bodies. A post-qualification training for staff working with people who present special challenges or difficult behavior which will integrate course work and supervised practice to achieve hands-on competence started in January, 1989.

Quality Assurance

Two hundred staff have been trained in Program Analysis of Service Systems (PASS), an evaluation tool focusing on the principle of normalization. A training package in quality assurance has been drafted and some parts have been piloted prior to region-wide introduction.

Evaluation And Research

Some evaluation of each of the training initiatives is an integral part of the work. For example, there have been follow-up surveys on the impact of the staffed housing course. Two larger projects are currently under way, one focusing on staff turnover in different types of mental handicap services and the other on the quality of life of people living in services. These projects have been set up with the special development team, using observable measures of individual activity both before and after transfer.

Mid-Essex Health Authority has appointed an Employee Development Advisor, whose role will be to clarify the implications for staff of service planning proposals. General managers in the authority will be encouraged to give staff training a much higher priority than it has hitherto been accorded. In 1986, a strategy for change was developed from two workshops involving senior managers and medical consultants. It identified themes for organizational change to make general management more workable, which included:

- The development of a corporate image and better public relationships;
- The need to be more user-oriented; the development of a clearer understanding of the relationship between user needs and demands and the resources available to the authority;

- Improvements to quality of service;
- The encouragement of greater innovation in service delivery accompanied by optimum delegation of decision-making;
- The need to build on organizational strengths against fairly pervasive national gloom about the National Health Service; and
- Improvements in internal communications and the development of better internal mechanisms for the resolution of conflict.

To implement the strategy for change successfully, it was vital not only to equip managers for what were, in many cases, new roles, but also to ensure their commitment to, and knowledge about, the necessary organizational changes. It was important to provide clear linkages between planned organizational and managerial development.

Eighty-two per cent of the senior and middle managers attended one of six core workshops. The district general manager, introducing each workshop, emphasized his commitment to management development and his expectations of managers. The rationale for personal effectiveness was that anyone who wants to improve the way he or she manages others must first learn self-management.

Workshop outcomes were articulated in terms of personal and organizational action planning. Personal planning enabled individuals to select further workshops on the basis of a diagnosis of personal development needs undertaken both individually and with peers during the initial workshop. Organizational planning involved the feedback of views on the nature and pressures of managerial roles as part of the continual evolution and implementation of the strategy of change. The latter data, together with subsequent evaluation letters from participants, enabled the management board to assess the degree to which the workshop's aims were met to set further goals of organizational change.

Six months later, participants attended a half-day activity at which individual action plans were reviewed and further blocks to individual and organizational development identified. The three-day core workshop program and the subsequent half-day follow-up cost approximately 10,000 pounds (British currency) plus about 25 days of senior management time. Administrative support was provided from within the organization.

Kent County Council Social Services Department is establishing fifteen community mental health teams. They are working with consultants from Birmingham and London Universities to develop appropriate training programs for these teams, which will include induction team workshops to establish a common philosophy, policy, and objectives and to further training in management, practice, and evaluation skills. Health service personnel and staff members of voluntary agencies will also participate. In addition, the training program will include public education sessions. The objective is to integrate planning and training in a combined program from its beginning. A four-day induction course was held which took as its theme the development of a comprehensive mental health service. Staff were then requested to begin thinking about the preparation of their area plans and the components of the service they wished to develop. A survey carried out prior to the beginning of the training had established the current baseline of existing services so everyone knew the point from which they were starting. The teams were issued a common format for the preparation of their plans.

A week-long block of training then followed as staff brought back their embryo plans for consultation. They had to produce immediate, interim, and long-term objectives within a specified framework. Running concurrently with this planning exercise was the training element designed to equip the new mental health managers with background knowledge and skills relevant to their management and development roles.

After a further two months of planning in the workplace, final formats were submitted to the development officer at headquarters. A detailed analysis of all the components contained in the six plans followed, and these were converted into the first draft of a county plan. Everyone had made a contribution to the overall plan, and it was hoped that this would achieve a sense of common ownership.

Central Norfolk Adult Education Department and Norwich Health Authority have devised a program in which staff and patients work together on issues raised by the transition to community services. Although the program has not yet started because of financial restraints, the ideas are interesting and worth describing here. For many people living in hospitals, this will have been the nearest thing they have known to home for much of their adult lives. As a result, people may experience a deep sense of loss when finding themselves in new and unfamiliar surroundings outside the hospital. Staff may also feel the effects of such changes in their working lives. Many of them will identify closely with the institution to which they will have committed so much time and energy over the years. Everyone engaged in this change of style and pace will need a period of adjustment and reflection.

The training program is innovative in that it seeks to link the process of redefinition of patients as adult learners with the changing roles of nurses as facilitators of community living. The project envisions the adult education authority working initially with nursing staff on a joint project through which staff development will be promoted. Adult education tutors would work with nurses and paramedical professionals to develop individual learning programs for a number of long-stay residents identified by ward and clinical teams.

The objectives of the program are as follows:

- To create a climate in which residents and staff will be able to make a smooth transition to life in the community.
- To assess daily living activities and/or personal interests of members of the care groups which might provide the focus for the development of a learning program.
- To identify realistic learning goals and activities compatible with the assessment stated above.

- To encourage all staff working with members of the care group to see their own relationship with the residents from the perspective of the residents as learners.
- To provide opportunities for staff to take part in off-the-job training with particular emphasis on the changing perspective of the work in which they are involved.

Alongside these examples, a number of other districts are developing pioneer concepts in some aspects of their training for community-based services. Sheffield Health Authority has a reorientation program for nursing staff, which is supported by organizational development work with the management group. The Mental Illness Unit of North East Essex Health Authority has created its own training plan which embraces basic and post-basic professional training; basic skills training; communication skills; induction and orientation sessions; an organizational development program; management training opportunities; staff appraisal; and general education. Training models such as these hopefully can point the way to more effective services and modalities for community mental health care in the future.

Notes

1. D. Braisby, et al., *Changing Futures: Housing and Support Services for People Discharged from Psychiatric Hospitals* (London: King Edward's Hospital Fund for London, 1988); D. Towell, "Health and Social Services Relationships in the reform of Long-Term Care," *British Journal of Social Work* 15 (1985); D. Towell and A. Davis, "Moving Out from the Large Hospitals: Involving the People (Staff and Patients) Concerned," *Care in the Community: Keeping it Local*, a report of MIND's 1983 annual conference, (London: MIND, 1984), 21–24; D. Towell and T. McAusland, eds., "Managing Psychiatric Services in Transition," *Health and Social Service Journal* 94 [center supplement] (October 18, 1984).

2. J. O'Brien, *The Principle of Normalization: A Foundation for Effective Services*, (adapted for CMH by Alan Tyne), (London: Campaign for Mentally Handicapped People, 1981); W. Wolfensberger, *The Principle of Normalization in Human Services* (Toronto: National Institute on Mental Retardation, 1972).

3. National Association for Mental Health (MIND), *Common Concern: MIND's Manifesto for a Comprehensive Mental Health Service* (London: MIND, 1983).

4. E. Kingsley, et al., *Up to Scratch: Monitoring to Maintain Standards* (London: King's Fund College, 1986), (unpublished paper).

5. D. Towell and S. Kingsley, *Developing Psychiatric Services in the Welfare State* (Psychiatric Services in Transition Paper No. 1), (London: King's Fund College, 1986).

6. See reference 1.

7. H. Smith, *Collaboration for Change: Partnership between Service Users, Planners and Managers of Mental Health Services* (KFC on 87/140). (London: King's Fund Centre, 1988).

8. Department of Health and Social Security. "Collaboration between the NHS, Local Government and Voluntary Organizations," (Health Circular/Local Authority Circular Draft). (London: DHSS, 1986).

9. National Federation of Housing Associations and MIND. *Housing: the Foundation of Community Care* (London: NFHA, 1987).

10. Audit Commission for Local Authorities—England and Wales, "Making a Reality of Community Care," (London: HMSO, 1986).

11. D. Andrews and H. Zutshi, Housing Support (Team Occasional Paper No. 1). "Training for Transition," (London: North Lambeth Day Centre, 1985).

12. Ibid.

13. M. Pedler, "Learning in Management Education," in: T.H. Boydell, *A Guide to the Identification of Training Needs*, 2nd ed. (London: British Association for Commercial and Industrial Education, 1976).

14. L. Ward and I. Wilkinson, eds. "Training for Change: Staff Training for 'An ordinary life'," (London: King Edward's Hospital Fund for London, 1985).

15. W.G. Perry, *Forms of Intellectual and Ethical Developments in the College Years* (London: Holt, Rinehart and Winston, 1970).

16. Further details of PASS and PASS Training Workshops are available from: CMH/CMHERA, 12a Maddox St, London W1 and MIND Training and Education Department, 22 Harley St, London W1.

17. W. Wolfensberger, *The Principle of Normalization in Human Services* (Toronto: National Institute on Mental Retardation, 1972).

18. B. Stocking, ed., *In Dreams Begins Responsibility: A Tribute to Tom Evans* (London: King Edward's Hospital Fund for London, 1987).

19. T. Peters and R.H. Waterman, *In Search of Excellence: Lessons from America's Best-Run Companies* (New York: Harper and Row, 1982).

20. Unpublished correspondence with Dr. T. Wainwright, Camberwell Health Authority (London, 1987).

21. N.V. Raynes, "Managing before Training: A Cautionary Tale in Care in the Community," *Hospital and Health Services Review* 83 (1987), 114–16.

22. J. Mansell, "Training for Service Development," in: D. Towell, ed. *An Ordinary Life in Practice: Developing Comprehensive Community-Based Services for People with Learning Difficulties* (London: King Edward's Hospital Fund for London, 1988), 129-40.

23. See reference 14.

24. See reference 14.

25. J. Mansell, et al: "Bringing People Back Home: South East Thames Regional Health Authority's Staff Training Initiative in Mental Handicap," (Bristol: National Health Service Training Authority).

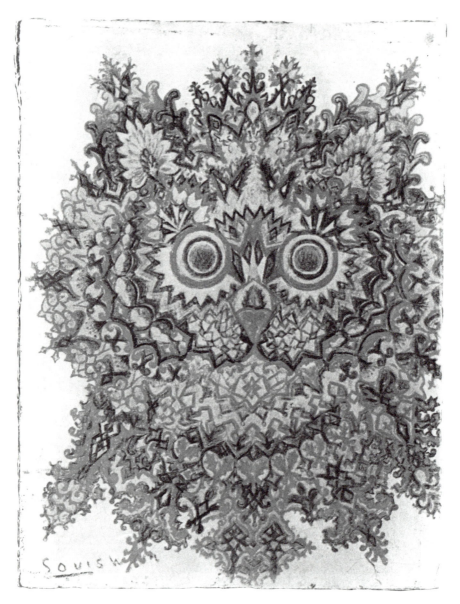

Decorative Representation of a Cat. Louis Wain, 20th Century; Art and History Collections, The Bethlem Royal Hospital, Kent, England.

MENTAL HEALTH SELF-ADVOCACY IN THE UNITED KINGDOM

By *Peter Campbell*

In the United Kingdom during the 1980s, the concepts of advocacy and self-advocacy gained some prominence in discussions of health and social services provision. In services for people with learning difficulties or those diagnosed as mentally ill, the advocacy issues have commonly become part of informed debate about the future shape of services.

Defining Advocacy And Self-Advocacy

An advocate is someone with particular skills who speaks and/or acts on behalf of another person or persons lacking such skills. With the development of health and social services, in recent decades, certain people or groups of people are perceived to be so significantly disadvantaged that they are unable to represent themselves in stating their desires, needs, grievances, and goals. As a result of this perception, different groups of workers in British services often attempt to act as advocates for their clients during the course of their everyday work. From this base, more specialized forms of advocacy have developed, such as legal advocacy and citizen advocacy. Legal advocates have professional skills which they make available to those whose cause they are pursuing. The citizen advocate may have no special expertise but he or she volunteers for training in establishing a relationship with an individual or small group of people in order to represent them and their concerns. There is wide acceptance for the idea that some people may be unable to present their own cases and, therefore, should have special assistance.

Self-advocacy should be the matrix which holds the various types of advocacy together. If individuals or groups who do not need specialized help in presenting their cases are being discouraged or prevented from doing so, then the whole structure of advocacy and its provision becomes irrelevant. Supportive facilities should be working toward the goal of self-advocacy; however, in the United Kingdom, advocacy both as concept and reality seems to have developed somewhat in advance of self-advocacy.

In examining self-advocacy as part of the British mental health self-advocacy movement, it is important to be aware of the distinction between individual and collective self-advocacy. The concept of an individual speaking or acting on his/her own behalf is central; but when groups of current and former service recipients work together to present their viewpoints, change the systems of psychiatric provision, and dispel social prejudice, this acts as a collective enterprise. The term, recipient/user action, indicates the direction of the movement more clearly than the term, self-advocacy.

In continuing to use the term self-advocacy, one needs to be aware of its limitations. In the British context, self-advocacy encompasses a wide range of activities, some of which are either loosely interconnected or contradictory. Action by recipients and recipient groups is a comparatively new phenomenon which does not always appear coherent to outside observers and analysts. In particular, it would be a serious mistake to consider the mental health self-advocacy movement in the United Kingdom as relevant only to service provision. Although there has been a significant response from service providers which has influenced the scope of action, recipient groups are not merely interested in achieving good services. Recipient groups are aiming for a change in social attitudes, and an alteration of the devalued personal and social status which adheres to the group currently defined as mentally-ill. Any understanding which fails to reflect this wide perspective is flawed.

Mental health self-advocacy is about empowerment in personal and social contexts. One of the major issues that remains to be confronted in the next few years in the United Kingdom is the degree to which such an approach can be reconciled with the positions currently expressed by the higher levels of health and social services establishments. At present it is, perhaps, sufficient to ask how the concepts of self-advocacy, as understood by the recipients active in the field, connect with ideas such as consumerism in the National Health Service, consultation, democratic representation, services based on individual need, and value for the money. It is in areas such as these that the future direction of recipient action and the quality of mental health service provision will be decided.

Origins And Current Position Of Mental Health Self-Advocacy In The United Kingdom

Ever since the middle of the 19th century with the creation of the asylum system and the establishment of the psychiatric profession, there has been a tradition of protest by and on behalf of those who found themselves being described and treated as mentally-ill. Such protest, evident in the 19th century in groups like the Alleged Lunatics Friend Society, has continued to the present day, achieving particular notoriety in the late 1960s in the anti-psychiatry movement associated with such figures as Thomas Szasz, R.D. Laing, and David Cooper. This movement, however, in spite of producing the Mental Patients' Union in Great Britain, failed to produce long-lasting or widespread action by recipients. It has only been in the last five years that significant action by independent groups of recipients has started to develop.

In 1985, at the time of the International Mental Health Charter 2000 Conference held in Britain, there were five or six independent action groups in the United Kingdom. There are now between 35 and 40 groups. A national umbrella organization called Survivors Speak Out tries to improve communication and contact among groups and individuals. Even though it does not act as a national voice, it promotes the idea of recipient action by combining the efforts of recipients, mental health workers, and the wider society. Although the number of people actively involved remains comparatively small, the changes that have already taken place are highly significant.

Mental health self-advocacy groups vary considerably in character as well as in their goals. All groups are devoted to promoting the viewpoint of the recipient. Many involve people such as mental health workers who are not recipients of services. Not all groups accord equal status to non-recipients in terms of voting or being on the group's executive committee, but the overall theme is one of partnership, not one of separation. The groups which currently exist can be loosely placed into the following categories:

- Groups closely associated with or involved in organizing existing service provisions;
- Groups devoted to establishing patients' councils and advocacy schemes within institutions, such as psychiatric hospitals or day care facilities;
- Local action groups operating in a range of ways to improve service provision and public attitudes within a particular locality; and
- Regional or national campaigning groups acting on issues such as the misuse of major tranquilizers.

Even after some years of successful activity, the majority of groups still have only minimal funding and little technical support or administrative back-up. In the last nine months, there have been a few signs that significant funding may become move available, but many groups are seriously over-extended and under-resourced. The next two years will be crucial in influencing the shape and future direction of mental health self-advocacy.

Three Examples Of Mental Health Self-Advocacy Groups

Nottingham
In the Nottingham area, there has been a pioneering attempt to introduce advocacy and self-advocacy facilities modeled on those developed in Holland. The Nottingham Patients' Council Support Group (NPCSG) and Nottingham Advocacy Group (NAG) have acted as models for various other areas of the United Kingdom, such as Brighton, Newcastle, and Leeds. The facilities being developed in Nottingham include patients' councils in three psychiatric hospitals, facilitated by NPCSG; a citizen's advocacy project run by NAG; the Dale Center, which is a day facility in the community largely organized by recipients; and recipient advo-

cacy groups in local areas of the city of Nottingham linked to statutory sector terms. There are plans to establish an independent legal advocate to work in the psychiatric hospitals. The objective is to ensure that recipients within the institutions and those living in the community can present their cases regardless of their ability to act for themselves.

Although overall progress has been encouraging in the Nottingham area, opposition and apathy towards the work of NPCSG and NAG has been a frequent hurdle to overcome. Within the psychiatric hospitals, the task of building a patients' council structure based on representation from patients-only meetings in each hospital ward has proved exceptionally difficult. Until this year, the work of NPCSG has been entirely based on volunteer efforts. Suspicion and hostility from ward staff have sometimes been surmounted, but often senior management reneges on promises to attend the meetings. When meetings have been attended by senior staff, however, the patients have sometimes been treated in a token manner, making progress even more difficult. Nevertheless, as a result of work in the last five years, Nottingham does now have the framework for a comprehensive system of advocacy and self-advocacy which could eventually provide the type of climate and the quality of services which many recipients are now seeking. The recent provision of funding for a full-time worker in support of NPCSG is a welcome boost to the development of the patients' council in both Nottingham and the nation.

Camden
Camden Consortium was founded in 1984, largely as a response from senior mental health workers to the closure plans for the local psychiatric hospital. It quickly developed into a local action group to promote the viewpoints of recipients with a particular focus on involving them in the planning of health and local authority mental health services. The group pursues a range of activities, including consciousness raising, campaigning and pressure group action, providing representatives to health and social services planning committees, and producing written material relating to services and recipients' experience.

The group's major piece of work to date was centered around a report entitled "Mental Health Priorities in Camden as We See Them—the Consumer Viewpoint," which was launched in June 1986. This report was based on questionnaires and workshops involving recipients within Camden and concentrated on three areas—acute crisis services, housing, and employment. Later, the Consortium developed specific proposals from this report on the need for a 24-hour crisis resource. This has led directly to the group's central involvement in current health and social services consideration of such a crisis provision.

The consortium has been particularly successful in producing written material. "Treated Well? A Code of Practice for Psychiatric Hospitals," produced with the help of Good Practices in Mental Health 1988, was an attempt to evaluate a service which has had a national impact from a recipient's perspective. The group's concern to be involved in the planning process has also been important. As a result, the consortium has achieved a position of regular involvement and consultation and now faces the problem of meeting a demand to provide representatives to nearly twenty different organizations and committees.

London

The London Alliance for Mental Health Action (LAMHA) is a combination of recipients, workers, volunteers, and trade union groups. It functions within the London area as a campaigning organization and has taken the lead in highlighting the perspective of recipients on a number of national mental health issues. While many mental health self-advocacy groups in the United Kingdom have developed significant involvement within the structures of service provision, LAMHA is not involved in providing representation on planning groups or other committees and it takes a radical campaigning position on issues of local and national concern.

LAMHA was created as a vehicle for coordinating opposition to proposals to alter the 1983 Mental Health Act and compels treatment of people in the community. The Compulsory Treatment Order (CTO) issue was a major feature of mental health debate in the United Kingdom in 1987–1988. The extension of compulsory powers still remains a real possibility. LAMHA ran an effective campaign to counter the pressures for such a change, including a street demonstration in London by recipients on an exclusively mental health issue. The anti-CTO campaign was followed by a partially successful attack on the use of negative stereotypes of schizophrenics in an advertising campaign by SANE (Schizophrenia: A National Emergency).

Although the trend within mental health self-advocacy in the last two or three years has been away from large-scale campaigning on major issues like compulsory powers in mental health care and the use of major tranquilizers, LAMHA remains an example of a particular line of action which may become more prominent in the near future as the idea of recipient action gains wider credibility at local and national levels.

The Future Of Mental Health Self-Advocacy

It is difficult to assess the achievements of mental health self-advocacy in the United Kingdom. One problem is to find acceptable criteria to use in an evaluation. In terms of actual units of service provision which have been substantially modified through recipient action, the evidence may be hard to find. In terms of opportunities for dialogue or improved attitudes towards recipients, the evidence is much greater. What should be remembered is that prior to 1985, there was virtually no recipient involvement, let alone empowerment. Whatever the limitations of current actions, tokenism is still more common than genuine collaboration or partnership. It would have been inconceivable to most recipients in the early 1980s. From the perspective of recipients, the achievement has been quite startling.

The major questions for the future must focus on the relationship between recipient action groups and the system of service provision. How will the service providers' desires for services well-matched to individual needs of consumers link with the recipient activists' demands for empowerment? There is already a range of postures being adopted by both parties. Large-scale and long-term involvement in the detailed planning and monitoring of services is one possibility. But the independent provision of services or criticism of state systems is another position which mental health self-advocacy groups could adopt. Although the recipient movement in the United Kingdom is not marked by the separatism which characterizes sections of the movement in the United States, it is quite possible that the provision of recipient-controlled services and political and legalistic campaigning on an organized scale, not yet very evident in the United Kingdom, will become more common in the future.

At present, there is insufficient evidence available to recipient groups to allow clear judgments about the effectiveness of particular strategies. Most contact with planners and managers is characterized by a mixture of genuine concern and a feeling that there will be severe limitations on sharing of power. Cooption, or committee action, rather than formal partnership, still remains a likely result of involvement within the service systems. On the other hand, participation in the other areas where decisions are made seems to make in-roads on isolation and non-involvement.

Great uncertainty currently characterizes mental health service provision in the United Kingdom. This is reflected in the area of mental health self-advocacy. As plans proceed to implement the changes recommended in the white paper, "Caring for People," there is increasing talk about user involvement. At this point there is very little evidence of serious thought about how this is going to happen, or serious attention to the right to advocacy and self-advocacy. The proposed changes to systems of service delivery may allow more choice and may even, in the long term, enable recipients to provide services for themselves. However, there are real fears that recipients will remain powerless in their dealings with service systems and that their position within society will not be altered at all.

For a variety of reasons, both recipient activists and service providers remain unclear about what they can achieve, as well as about the intentions and activities of each other. It is important that greater clarity and honesty be quickly achieved. It is increasingly evident that recipient groups cannot continue to survive and undertake effective work unless they are properly funded. If groups with funds—government departments, health authorities, or national voluntary groups—are going to make money available, they should make that fact clear and then indicate the conditions they will attach to granting it. If government intentions and recipient actions are incompatible, which in present circumstances seems entirely possible, the sooner it is acknowledged the better.

There is still an enormous imbalance of power among the parties involved. However confused or divided the systems of service provision are, they still have the ability to divert or devour the efforts of those involved in mental health self-advocacy. If mental health self-advocacy is valued, more thought must be given to allowing it to develop in its own fashion and more detailed consideration must be given to supporting that development in a practical way. Otherwise, there is a very real danger that recipient action's potential to ameliorate inadequate services and to transform public attitudes and sympathies will dissolve into a bland, easily-managed mental health market consumerism.

∿ FINANCING CARE OF THE CHRONIC MENTALLY ILL

By Peter Kennedy, MD

When planning mental health services and targeting money, the chronic mentally ill (CMI) figure most prominently in the minds of the public, politicians, managers, and professionals. Nevertheless, everything seems to conspire to direct the money elsewhere or exclude the CMI from the very services provided. The parties concerned may blame each other, but usually each is responsible in one way or another. Usually, the mentally ill themselves are the scapegoats. Their needs are so changeable that they do not conform to obvious patterns and tend to slip from view.

Having a clear understanding of how this perverse process develops is the surest way to build in preventive safeguards. Everyone concerned should know the traps and tricks that take money away from where it was intended. They should watch each other carefully and promptly call individuals to account.

The Dowry From The Mental Hospital

Mental hospitals were designed and built for the younger CMI adult. It seems reasonable, therefore, that money for the community care of these individuals should be realized from these hospitals as they gradually empty. Figure 1 shows graphs of declining bed use in mental hospitals in York, a fairly typical mental health service with a population of around 600,000. It shows that from 1975, when systematic recording began, there was a steady decline in bed occupancy as the old, long-term patients died off and the younger chronically mentally ill were discharged or not allowed to become long-term residents. This trend was determined by clinicians acting in the best interests of their patients without government policy to instruct them. However, up to the mid-1980s, hardly any money was released from the mental hospitals which meant that more patients in the community were sharing a lower allocation of support. The objection to closing one of the three mental hospitals in York, as well as wards in the other hospitals, was that money should be invested in improved community care before reducing these facilities. As a result, professional staff were unwittingly diverting money from these patients either to finance useless spare capacity in the hospitals or to increase the quality of care for the residual hospital population. Aggregating patients and closing wards progressively, followed by closing whole hospitals or

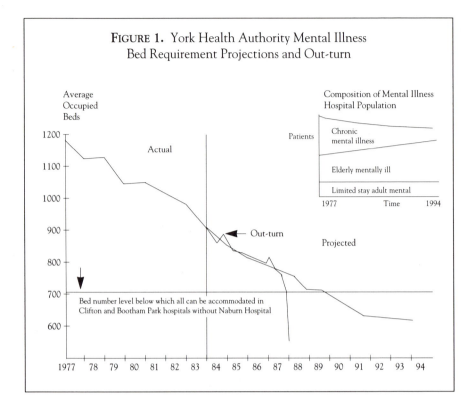

FIGURE 1. York Health Authority Mental Illness
Bed Requirement Projections and Out-turn

hospital blocks to release the fixed as well as the variable revenue costs, make the estate a saleable capital asset. Variable cost in nursing can be withdrawn as each ward closes, which represents about 60 percent of the cost of running a ward. When a block or hospital is closed, the remaining 40 percent becomes available from fixed costs in maintenance, services, and administration.

In York, as soon as everyone understood that resistance to closing wards was depriving the CMI of care financed by substantial revenue and capital, the pace of change accelerated and the closure of Naburn Hospital occurred before its projected target date. However, a fear remains that large sums of money released from the mental hospital closure will disappear without a clear plan for its reinvestment in community services. In fact, there is plenty of justification for this fear, and it is the responsibility of mental health professionals to make sure that sound financial plans for the CMI are drawn up early to make proper use of revenue and capital released from such mental hospitals.

There are two common errors that keep money from patients. The first is deferring closure, blaming government and the region for lack of enabling funds. Actually, imaginative brokerage with other districts and partial land sales of mental hospital sites before they are fully vacated can bridge this gap at the local level. The second is the mistake of funding community care of discharged patients on an average cost-per-case basis. This usually means spending far too much on those with lesser disabilities who are discharged early in the program, leaving far too little for the more disabled whose care incurs much higher-than-average cost.

Knapp and Leff report a range of costs per case of patients discharged from Friern Hospital from 47 to 568 pounds (British currency) per week. This study is starting to counter the myth that community care of the CMI will cost a great deal more than the cost of their care in the institution. Research psychiatrists Knapp and Leff report that provision of services in the community can be cheaper and better as far as measurement of mental state symptomatology and social functioning are concerned.

The Target Population

It is not just the misappropriation of mental health funds for acute services that has to be watched, it is also the extent to which money previously invested in long-term residential care for the CMI is unwittingly transferred to care of the elderly mentally ill or into acute psychiatry where the majority of patients being treated do not have a chronic condition. Figure 1 shows that in York, as the long-term patient population in the hospital declined and the chronic population in the community increased, funds shifted towards caring for the increasing numbers of elderly senile patients in the hospital.

In collaboration with Professor David Goldberg of the Department of Psychiatry at Manchester University, research scientist Kate Wooff demonstrated that funds put into community care to employ more community nurses, with care of the CMI as a priority, were soon diverted to other purposes.[2] These community psychiatric nurses gave increasingly less time to the support and care of the chronic schizophrenic and more time to counseling and crisis intervention for neurotics, the bereaved, and other patients with relatively minor psychiatric morbidity who had been referred by general practitioners. Day centers and community mental health centers, established to meet the needs of chronic patients discharged from mental hospitals, show similar patterns. Chronic patients often assist by not turning up and not complaining so that the withdrawal of funds and services from them goes unnoticed.

Retaining expensive professional services is one important reason why community services for the CMI become detached from the very people they are supposed to serve. The table in Figure 2 shows the components of the costs of caring for the CMI discharged from Friern Hospital. This shows that the proportion of the average cost actually required for a psychiatric nurse or psychiatrist is very small. It is inevitable that if a larger proportion of the funds coming out of mental hospitals has already inflated such professional staff, they will find work to do—not with the CMI but with other groups who can engage their skills more intensively.

FIGURE 2. Components of Costs Per Discharged Patient

	Pounds (British currency)
Total (Average)	270 per week
Housing and Living	209
Day Care	27
Education	3
General Practitioner	1
Injections	1
Nurse	1
Psychiatrist	1
Social Worker	10
Hospital Stays	12
Other	5

(Table adapted from Knapp and Leff data on Friern Hospital)

According to the analysis in Figure 2, many mental health strategies may be excessive in one area, such as providing highly skilled professional services, and concurrently deficient in providing other services, such as those related to housing, day care, education, and social support. It is not surprising that these patients drift away from services which are not tailored to their needs.

Targeting Needs

Ever since Farris and Dunham published their classical study in 1939 on how chronic schizophrenics drift away from their parent culture to the isolation of big city centers, it has been easy to blame the nature of the disorder itself on the fact that community mental health services lose a lot of their clients. At least part of this process might be due to a lack of flexibility and imagination in designing services to meet the needs of these patients. It costs between 3,000 and 4,000 pounds (British currency) a year for a place in a mental health day center. Such individuals might have a more comfortable and enriched life if they could be given the 25 pounds-per-day cost to spend on better alternatives. This money would create opportunities for individuals and their families to relieve the boredom and tensions of life, allowing for more interesting pursuits otherwise unavailable to them because of unemployment and low income.

There are certain euphemisms like "difficult to place patient" or "patients with challenging behavior" that are used to describe the more difficult chronic patient. All sorts of rationalizations tend to come into play to get rid of them. Until financial systems really do ensure that money follows patients, there will always be reinforcement of non-essential rather than essential services. For those patients who do not go away, one solution is to establish an expensive special needs unit. If this means a high staff-patient ratio in a ward of average security level, then it can be a very inflexible solution. The numbers requiring this care are very small, and fluctuations in demand mean that it can be over-subscribed or empty from one month to the next. Because the resource is fixed, nothing is available for someone who doesn't need to be in a ward but needs a lot of care outside. An individual may be forced, by a compulsory order of the Mental Health Act, to submit to treatment because financing for his/her care in the community is unavailable.

It is a courageous service that decides it can do without such a facility. It will require a small multidisciplinary team of dedicated individuals to work together bringing the best expertise and the best ideas to bear on finding solutions for individual patients. An incentive that most mental health professionals have never had is the availability of significantly large sums of money, up to 1,000 pounds (British currency) per week per patient, when a very high level of care in the community is required. For example, a brain-damaged, psychotic, partially blind, very aggressive young man was cared for in the home of his elderly parents to the satisfaction of all concerned. A joint contingency fund for health and social services allowed the provision of personal care assistants seven days a week for prolonged exacerbations of his condition.

Flexible funding of this kind could be the stimulus for more imaginative individual care. However, flexible funding is only possible if large sums of money are not tied up in intensive care in-patient units.

The Safeguards

If the CMI are not to lose the money available for their needs, a whole series of safeguards must be built into the process of closing outdated institutional facilities. The amounts of revenue and capital to become available must be identified and secured before the closure process gets under way. The population of persons for whom this money is to be allocated needs to be described clearly. Explicit plans for spending capital and revenue must be developed. Money should be targeted to particular groups of patients rather than to particular facilities. Investment in facilities must be as flexible as possible to switch use as the needs of individual patients change and the aggregate needs of the group alter with time. There must be clear procedures for inclusion of new patients in the target group and for the withdrawal of resources from patients who no longer require them, all made on the basis of careful needs assessments.

The specific mental health grant proposed in the new community care white paper "Caring for People," is a good start. If it leads local health and social services to agree on budgets and what needs to be done for specific patients, it will go a long way toward delegation of decisions to the level where the needs of individuals are perceived most clearly. A computerized monitoring system is probably essential, which would include names of patients who are recipients of care from this fund along with clear criteria for the removal of patients from the register and the admission of new cases. There should be a requirement for periodic reassessments of need and early identification of the names of patients who have disappeared.

In the York Mental Health Service, with a monitoring system of this kind over a period of 18 months, just over 20 out of a total of 300 people with serious disabilities were untraceable. What is required to avoid perverse incentives for losing such individuals from a service is an agreement that when an itinerant person with CMI turns up in another area, requiring health and social services, the area of origin could be billed for the cost of that individual's care. Case managers would then have the incentive for doing their utmost to design a flexible service, responsive to the needs of individuals, rather than simply writing off money from their budgets when clients go elsewhere.

It can be an intricate business to oversee money for the CMI and ensure that those for whom it was intended continue to have access to it. Perhaps each district needs an advocate, who is independent of all statutory services but intimately involved in watching how mental health money is spent, to properly look after the needs of the CMI. It is a form of advocacy that is not likely to be difficult to implement. This individual could help to ensure that a specific mental health grant is rationed among defined patients. He or she would effectively counteract the inexorable tendency for such moneys to be used for other purposes. It is such impartial involvement and oversight that can bring gradual improvement to mental health self-advocacy in the United Kingdom.

Notes

1. M. Knapp and J. Leff, are research psychiatrists working for the Medical Research Council.
2. K. Wooff, D. Goldberg, and T. Fryers, "Patients in Receipt of Community Psychiatric Care in Salford," *Psychological Medicine* 16, 407–14.
3. R.G. Faris and H.W. Dunham, *Mental Disorders in Urban Areas* (Chicago: Hafner, 1939).